Back to a New Normal

In Search of Stability in an Era of Pandemic Disruption— Insight From Practitioners and Academics

Back to a New Normal

In Search of Stability in an Era of Pandemic Disruption—Insight From Practitioners and Academics

Edited by

S. Charles Malka
Sullivan University

and

Robert H. Tiell
Psychology Resource Group

IAP

Information Age Publishing, Inc.
Charlotte, North Carolina • www.infoagepub.com

Library of Congress Cataloging-in-Publication Data

CIP data for this book can be found on the Library of Congress website:
http://www.loc.gov/index.html

Paperback: 978-1-64802-821-2
Hardcover: 978-1-64802-822-9
eBook: 978-1-64802-823-6

Printed and bound by CPI Group (UK) Ltd, Croydon, CR0 4YY

In loving memory of my father, Jacob Malka (1925–2020)

In loving memory of my parents,
Blanche Tiell (1918–1998) and Irvin Tiell (1910–1972),
and my mentor Dave Dobson (1915–1978)

CONTENTS

ACKNOWLEDGMENTS

This edited book could not have been completed without the contributions of our authors. They have been a superb group of academics and practitioners with a collective work experience, wisdom and knowledge that spans several decades. They answered our call in short order, and were up to the challenge of helping illuminate various aspects of the dark pandemic, and offer expert advice for remediating its effects. Above all, their timely and meaningful contributions promise to better prepare us for the post-COVID-19 era, and for future pandemics that are likely to erupt.

We also thank Anthony M. Zipple, chief problem solver, Silverflux Solutions, Michael Gritton, executive director of KentuckianaWorks, Lisa Willner, PhD, member, Kentucky House of Representatives, and past executive director of the Kentucky Psychological Association, for believing in the promise of this book, and in the message found within its pages.

Back to a New Normal: In Search of Stability in an Era of Pandemic Disruption—Insight From Practitioners and Academics, p. xi

PREFACE

A year into the pandemic, more than 100 million individuals have been infected with COVID-19, and more than 3.2 million worldwide have died. In the United States alone, 30 million have been infected and over 550,000 Americans succumbed to the pandemic. The global rollout of vaccines promises to reduce related infections and mortality rates, but epidemiologists warn that COVID is less likely to disappear compelling the world to coexist with the virus much like the seasonal flu. This prediction is supported by the ease with which the virus spreads, by the new mutations that continuously generate new strains, and by the fact that large parts of the world may remain behind with little or no access to vaccines. Should these processes continue, their combined effects may turn COVID-19 into an endemic. Namely, the virus remains persistent and manageable but requires periodic vaccination. Such development may also preserve the newly adopted practices at work and at home; social distancing may continue along with remote working, remote learning, masking and testing. We may gain back some measure of normality, but it is likely to be a new normal.

Overcoming the virus may provide a respite from its immediate effects but not from the long-term devastating impact on human life and world economies. Human and material losses cannot be swept away nor forgotten. Remembering COVID's harmful consequences helps the community of nations better prepare for the next pandemic that may be more severe. It requires keeping in mind the lessons that COVID has taught us, and be cognizant of the developments and changes it introduced as well as the costs it exerted beyond the sheer loss of human life. The pandemic damaged world economies and caused a severe global recession. It triggered

Back to a New Normal: In Search of Stability in an Era of Pandemic Disruption—Insight From Practitioners and Academics, pp. xiii–xviii

massive layoffs, prompted business closings, disrupted supply chains, and resulted in shortages in products and services.

The tectonic shifts induced by COVID affect us in many ways and not the least of which is how we now use digital tools for work, learning, worship and play; with the change in employment patterns and the swelling of the gig economy; with social isolation to which many are exposed; with the increased blurring of work-life lines; with the changes in travel and entertainment patterns; and with the redefinition of medical care. It may take time to accurately assess the impact these changes will have on individuals and on organizations. Yet, there is a growing consensus as to the need for families to better balance their work-school-home responsibilities in light of the relocation of virtual school and work to the living room. And, for employers to be more attuned to employees needs and health concerns.

The corona virus pandemic has propelled us to rethink the way we interact with others both at home and at work. Weighing related risks at work and school compelled individuals to adapt to remote working and learning cognitively and attitudinally, and adopt new behaviors. Organizations are forced to redefine their external and internal boundaries and practices in the way they interact with other organizations and with their own employees. For one, how to effectively manage and properly incentivize the work force has become a top priority for employers large and small. This necessitates a reconsideration of the role and importance of HR in strategically managing the company's human capital.

Indeed, new opportunities have also sprung up that carry implications for the way we live, work and travel. Consider, for instance, that COVID-19 fueled growth in some industries such as pharmaceuticals, at-home testing, protective gear, and diagnostic equipment makers. Artificial Intelligence applications may experience widespread use led by manufacturers who are likely to accelerate automation; automation ensures less workforce disruptions caused by social distancing thus reducing the number of employees on assembly lines. Airports and airlines are likely to operate vaccine passport systems as a condition for future travel. And aside from such trends, the pandemic also exposed new needs that call for innovative solutions, personal initiative and adaptation as the following handful of examples suggest.

- Remote learning and remote working increased demand for digital tools and related applications both at home and at the workplace. This, in turn, has created unmet demand for chips further straining global supplies of components across electronic devices. At the same time, it also opened up opportunities for innovative products. One such product is Viva, a new Microsoft application designed to address remote work related challenges, such as the fragmentation of human resource-based applications and the need for all-encompassing employee management systems. Viva is a unified software package that is specifically designed for human resource management current needs triggered by the pandemic (Torry, 2021).

- Remote work and remote learning exposed shortcomings inherent in current desktops and laptops. Computer companies are busy upgrading the quality of cameras and sound systems as well as tightening security and privacy needs that better meet the demands in the new work-from-home, and study-from-home era. Redesigned hardware promises to have better screens, improved noise control, rich virtual backgrounds, and better wireless connections that ultimately make us look better and sound better on our digital tools.
- Touchless payment technology has been adopted by more people since the pandemic hit. A prime reason is the desire of many consumers to avoid touching bills and coins as a potential carrier of the corona virus. According to the U.S Department of Commerce, digital retail sales were up 37% in third quarter of 2020, reducing cash payment as an option (Torry, 2021).
- The pandemic compelled parents to take charge and adopt a hands-on approach with their children's schooling. The shift to home schooling is one expression of parents' frustration with school closings and the sporadic remote learning. Experts contend that children's home schooling may lead to the proliferation of options beyond public or private education. Just how widespread is the current shift to home schooling? Consider, for instance, that North Carolina's home-monitoring website crashed on the first day of enrollment, and close to 20,000 families elected to file for home schooling from July 2020 to January 2021, double the filing from an earlier year (Bauerlein, 2021).
- Faced with forced layoffs and employment uncertainties brought about by the pandemic, many have decided to take control of their own employment by joining the gig economy as freelancers. Toptal is a freelancing website that links companies and freelance workers with experience and expertise in desired fields. Toptal reported that between March 2020 and early January 2021, close to 300,000 freelancers registered for its website use (Smith, 2021). Such increase in numbers of freelancers suggests that COVID-19 accelerated business' shift toward the use of freelancers, thus legitimizing the gig economy as a whole.

The common thread that runs through these examples points to the opportunities that a crisis provides and to the human ingenuity and adaptation when dealing with unpredictable challenges. The lightning speed with which pharma companies took it upon themselves to develop vaccines is perhaps the most remarkable example of human ingenuity at its best. Promising results recorded in Israel, a country that led the world in per capita vaccinations, provide encouraging signs as to their effectiveness. A glimmer of hope is now shared by many experts in light of recent scientific and pharmaceutical breakthroughs, and advancements in new therapeutics. Additional reasons for a reserved optimism are proposed by healthcare experts. Consider that the recent mutations discovered in the United Kingdom, Brazil and South Africa appear to be under relative control. Note that the number of flu cases is surprisingly negligent given that we are in the midst of what otherwise would be the peak of a flu season. As critical, resistance to vaccination continues to level off and is now somewhat subdued in many countries. And not least important is the revolutionary mRNA molecule developed by Moderna that has been successful as a vaccine fighting various other viruses. The success rate of the molecule as a vaccine against COVID-19 reached 94.5% efficiency. And finally, consider the growth in a new related trend: remote medical intervention. Telemedicine is accelerating by using the internet as an alternative platform for addressing patients' health needs, thus ensuring less gathering of the sick in enclosed clinics.

And while hope is an important ingredient for the soul and spirit, so is the pressing need to surmount the pandemic-induced changes and challenges that we are confronted with. The pandemic challenges policy makers with the need to formulate and sponsor community-based programs that address health and employment related needs of individuals and families affected by the virus. One such area concerns the unemployed. Job search programs for the unemployed and particularly the long-term unemployed are vital for securing employment to millions of laid off workers. The pandemic also challenges researchers and practitioners in developing empirical-based and practical-based know-how for adequately addressing pressing questions worthy of exploration. For instance, when considering remote learning and remote work, many related questions are worth exploring.

- How to assess the effects of the pandemic on school children? Is virtual learning equally effective across all grades? Is there a difference in retention-absorption of learning content between synchronous and asynchronous methods? How to measure the impact of remote learning? What are some sound practices for remote learning? How can collaboration between teacher-student, and between student-student be enhanced? What are some of the strategies for managing the virtual classroom?

- How can companies facilitate remote work? What strategies can a company employ for reducing employee feelings of isolation? What must companies do for diffusing remote work related conflict? How can a company ensure employee productivity when working remotely? How should companies incentivize remote work? What should companies do to secure employee privacy and safeguard company secrets and intellectual property?
- What should workers do to remain motivated, organized, and productive? What must employees do to remain healthy when working remotely? Are there strategies that ensure a healthy balance of work-life responsibilities?
- How has the pandemic affected the well-being of at risk populations such as the elderly, the chronically ill, and members of other marginalized groups?
- What is the pandemic impact on the mental health and well-being of employees in particularly devastated industries such as hospitality, healthcare, travel and entertainment? What protections should be in place to mitigate risks of future pandemics?
- What changes has the pandemic imposed at the organization level with regard to new leadership roles, allocation of resources, strategic management of human capital, and crisis management?

Our preliminary list of questions may be far from complete. Notably, listed are questions that involve the relocation of work and learning to home settings, and to their effects and manifestation at both the personal and organizational levels. Many other questions are left open, while many more may surface by the time the virus is stopped. We attempted to tackle head-on a few of these questions. We are firm believers in exploring opportunities for change that COVID-19 opened up along with the lessons it taught us. For that purpose, we asked a group of experts from the academia and practitioners from various fields to share their know how and experience dealing with the consequences of the pandemic, and offer strategies for coping with its harmful effects. Our book follows in this vein.

Each one of the book chapters approaches the pandemic and its effects from a different angle, and in addition to exploring the dark side of the pandemic, opportunities for change are discussed along with practical strategies for dealing with some of the virus' disruptive consequences. If nothing else, the imposed changes in one's life also call for careful reflections on the new reality within which we are expected to work, learn, and play. Just how likely would it be for us to gather ourselves and walk back into the old way of doing things? Some believe we will simply return to our prepandemic *normal* world. On the other hand, our premise behind this book is that we may instead be on the threshold of a *new* normal. We believe that we should better prepare for it and for worse pandemics to come.

—S. Charles Malka and Robert H. Tiell
June 2021

REFERENCES

Smith, R. (2021, February 1). How to go freelance during the pandemic. *The Wall Street Journal*, p. A12.

Tilley, A. (2021, February 5). Microsoft CEO sees teach shift lasting. *The Wall Street Journal*, pp. B1, B2.

Torry, H. (2021, February 1). Cashless future? Don't bank on it. *The Wall Street Journal*, p. A2.

PART I

WORKFORCE AND WORKPLACE CHALLENGES AND OPPORTUNITIES

CHAPTER 1

INVISIBLE HEROES

The Mission Critical Role of HR During the COVID-19 Pandemic

Teresa A. Daniel

OVERVIEW

COVID-19 is the disease caused by a relatively new coronavirus called SARS-CoV-2. It was first discovered by the World Health Organization in late December of 2019, following a report of a cluster of cases of "viral pneumonia" in Wuhan, People's Republic of China (World Health Organization, 2020). The coronavirus was called "novel" because scientists had never seen it before. Along the way, experts have been surprised by its virulence, transmission, symptoms, impact on daily life, the magnitude of the sickness it causes, and the staggering death toll it has caused that continues to climb (Huang, 2021; Mineo, 2021).

The pandemic resulting from the widespread outbreak of this disease has caused serious mental, physical, and financial complications for people everywhere. It has been a devastating and disruptive global event—what some have referred to as a collective "mass trauma" (Prideaux, 2021) or a "shared tragedy" (Hamblin, 2021). The toll of the pandemic can be assessed by a variety of devastating metrics: hundreds of thousands of

Back to a New Normal: In Search of Stability in an Era of Pandemic Disruption—Insight From Practitioners and Academics, pp. 3–14

lives lost, millions of jobs eliminated, businesses permanently closed, hundreds of millions of school hours which took place at home with children working on a computer screen, and holidays, celebrations, and vacations canceled for most families during the year.

People and organizations have been forced to navigate a crisis of epic proportion for which there is no playbook. Radical changes to the workplace have elevated the profile of human resource (HR) practitioners during the past year (Devlin, 2021). Organizations are relying on them more than ever to keep workers safe, while also ensuring that they stay productive, committed, and engaged at work. As a profession, HR may be defined for generations by how we respond to this moment.

THE IMPACT OF THE PANDEMIC ON EMPLOYEES

Throughout most of the pandemic, employees have been expected to perform their normal work duties from home, while also trying to juggle competing roles as parent, teacher, and caregiver—24/7—with no opportunity for travel or vacation, and virtually no time off-duty. As a result, the boundaries of the typical workday that once separated work and home life blurred beyond recognition, frequently leaving employees feeling stressed, exhausted, disengaged, isolated, and underappreciated (Chawla et al., 2020).

Many employees have legitimately worried that simply going to the office could have deadly consequences. Similarly, *not* going to the office but being required to work from home clearly wreaked havoc on employee health and well-being too. Although the situation has been particularly acute for those employees with children whose schools were shut down (requiring them to learn from home), it is highly likely that single and childless workers have also been impacted due to increased feelings of loneliness, isolation from colleagues, and serious disruption to their day-to-day lives (Achor et al., 2018).

Equally troubling to most people was the absence of knowing when the pandemic would end or what the "new normal" would actually look like once it did. Reducing the "unknowns" is typically an important strategy for HR practitioners to adopt in order to make bad situations a bit more bearable for employees. In a constantly evolving situation like a global pandemic, though, solutions to complex problems tend to live in the realm of the unknown. The truth is that there have been no best practices for HR to follow because there has been no recent experience from which decision-makers could draw.

In a 2020 study of nearly 1,500 people from 46 countries (most of whom had worked remotely for at least part of the year), a team of burnout researchers explored the main issues that employees have faced during the pandemic. A staggering 85% of the participants reported the following:

- a decline in their general well-being and mental health;
- an increased and unsustainable workload;
- feelings of disengagement, isolation/lack of connection with colleagues; and
- home-life struggles.

In addition, they noted a lack of leader support, concerns about their job security, and difficulties meeting basic physical needs (Campbell & Gavett, 2021). They also reported a comparable decline in workplace well-being due to similar concerns (89%), and also included anxiety about changes to their day-to-day routines, new technology demands, and significant employment changes.

Not surprisingly, employees working in jobs with high physical proximity and frequent interaction (e.g., teachers in classrooms, leisure and travel venues (including restaurants and hotels), on-site customer interaction centers, computer-based office work, and production and warehousing were the most disrupted during the pandemic (McKinsey Global Institute, 2021). These are the occupations which are predicted to experience longer-lasting effects of the pandemic. For less dense workspaces (such as outdoor production sites), the effects of the pandemic are expected to fade more quickly.

THE CHANGING ROLE OF HR DURING THE PANDEMIC

The disruption caused by the pandemic is not limited to employees, though; it has also significantly changed the focus and role of HR professionals—while at the same time increasing their importance to the organization. They have been working around the clock, taking exceptional measures to keep employees safe and to ensure that their organizations survive.

During this time of crisis, HR practitioners have been meeting frequently with senior leaders, as well as health and safety experts, about how best to navigate this situation. They are the ones helping to keep employees informed about how the company plans to keep them safe when they physically return to work. HR has also been relentlessly communicating with employees about potential changes to their jobs (e.g., layoffs, pay cuts, benefit changes, etc.).

In partnership with senior leaders, they are updating policies and benefit programs that impact the lives of employees and their families. They are delivering bad news to employees as hard decisions are made about organizational changes required to keep the company in business. They have been developing remote work policies and helping employees adjust to the sudden changes to their day-to-day lives, both at home and at work (Smith, 2021a).

They are also developing guides and resource sites to help employees work effectively from home, meeting with anxious employees to provide emotional support, implementing strategies to keep employees engaged and committed, dealing with employees concerns about their use of new technologies required to operate virtually, developing new virtual strategies to recruit and on-board new hires, implementing new safety protocols to prevent the spread of germs in the office, and counseling with employees about their vaccination concerns (e.g., Bingham, 2020; Burrus, 2020; Grensing-Pophal, 2021; Smith, 2021b).

In addition, HR practitioners have also been required to implement many new and complex COVID-19 related laws and governmental regulations that have been issued to protect employees and their organizations (e.g., Families First Coronavirus Response Act [U.S. Department of Labor, 2020] which impacts employees or the Paycheck Protection Program [U.S. Small Business Administration, 2020–2021], or Coronavirus Aid, Relief, and Economic Security (CARES) Act [U.S. Department of the Treasury, 2020] which provide opportunities for business as a whole, among other governmental actions).

Although staying current with numerous regulations is not new to HR, what makes this situation different is that the laws and guidelines are being updated frequently as the science about COVID-19 continues to quickly evolve (Segal, 2021). This constant change is creating contradiction and confusion about which guidelines employers should actually follow in order to keep employees safe.

The changes caused by the pandemic have also resulted in an explosion of articles, toolkits, and policy guidance for HR professionals to read, much of it issued by the national Society for Human Resource Management (SHRM, n.d.). In fact, a portion of SHRM's website is now devoted to the accumulation of resources to help HR practitioners manage through the many complex workplace and legal issues related to COVID-19.

Many companies have implemented mask mandates as part of their safety protocols, but not all employees are in favor of such policies. They sometimes refuse or complain about having to wear this type of protective equipment. Given that mask-wearing has also become highly politicized (Huang, 2021), these situations are tricky to navigate. This is why practitioners have been called "organizational diplomats" when it comes to mask enforcement (Lumen, 2020). The decision whether or not to mandate COVID-19 vaccinations before employees return to work are likely to exacerbate this potentially conflictual situation further (Smith, 2021b). In addition, as we enter the late stages of the pandemic, practitioners are also being required to navigate the very real implications of "pandemic fatigue" as employees grow weary of the many restrictions imposed during the past year (Smith, 2021a).

There has also been an increased emphasis on technology issues as practitioners have determined that their current HR and workforce software cannot deliver the privacy and security that they require during the pandemic (Lumen, 2020). HR has historically been connected to the corporate network when working on systems containing sensitive employee data. With dispersed HR employees now disconnected from the more secure platform, the challenges for HR of ensuring privacy and security of sensitive health and other employee data have significantly increased.

Dealing with all of these rapid-fire changes would be difficult to manage under any circumstance, but it has been particularly hard this past year given that HR practitioners have had their own personal losses, concerns, and anxieties about the pandemic to deal with too.

ACCELERATION OF HR'S EMPLOYEE SUPPORT ROLE

Employees routinely bring emotionally-charge problems to HR with the expectation that they will receive help to resolve those issues or at least see someone who will listen to them. During these situations, HR practitioners have a very unique role—they operate as *organizational toxin handlers.*

Peter Frost (2003, 2004, 2006) first coined the term. Daniel (2017, 2018, 2020) extended the concept by finding that the function is actually a significant part of HR's role. When working in this capacity, toxin handlers provide emotional support by helping employees deal with difficult or painful emotions so that they can stay focused and productive.

With the COVID-19 pandemic, the economy in free fall, and difficult layoff and return-to-work decisions currently being made by organizations across the United States, this HR support is needed more than ever. Not only are employees reacting to difficult workplace decisions (e.g., pay cuts and job eliminations), but they are also juggling the very real stresses related to COVID-19 related illnesses and deaths—which may affect them personally or which may impact someone they love.

While working as a toxin handler, HR engages in six core activities: empathetic listening; suggesting solutions and providing resources; working behind the scenes to provide a secure place for employees to discuss their concerns; strategically communicating and reframing difficult messages; confidential counseling; as well as coaching and advising managers (Daniel, 2018). Serving in this capacity is a critical part of the HR role at all times, but toxin handlers are most especially important during times of crisis like the pandemic.

Without this organizational support from HR, employee stress and distraction would continue to build, resulting in higher levels of turnover, increased health costs, more litigation, more absences, and reduced levels of employee morale, well-being, and productivity. Although employees rely heavily on HR to provide this support, it is often invisible to the organization because most of these conversations, of necessity, are confidential and occur behind closed doors.

CHANGING ASSUMPTIONS ABOUT WORK

Once the pandemic ends, it would be prudent for HR practitioners to collectively take a pause. Instead of racing to return to "normal," we should take time to reflect on all that we have learned—about how and where employees work best, about the additional skills training that might be useful, and about what level of technology, resources, or travel is really required in order for employees to be productive and engaged—and then act rapidly and decisively to implement those desired changes before we forget them.

Several of the most pervasive beliefs about work have been: (1) that many jobs cannot be effectively performed remotely, (2) that employees cannot really be productive (whether at home or in the office) without a supervisor present to continuously monitor their work, and (3) that employees have someone at home to cover childcare and other day-to-day demands of life when schedules are abruptly changed, or travel is required without much advance notice. Moreover, the conventional wisdom prior to the pandemic was that meetings needed to occur in person to get anything done, that everyone be together in the same physical space in order to innovate and collaborate, that work relationships could not be sustained through video calls, and that business travel was an absolute necessity.

The reality of our collective experience during the pandemic has shattered these views and revealed them to be myths in most workplaces (e.g., Lindzon, 2021; Nintex, 2021; McKinsey Global Institute, 2021). We quickly learned that more work can be done remotely than we previously thought, including business sales calls, legal arbitration, judicial proceedings, doctor visits, classroom learning, and real estate tours. We also learned that some work that technically can be conducted remotely might actually be best accomplished in person—such as the schooling of young children and individuals with special needs, negotiations, providing sensitive feedback, and onboarding new employees (McKinsey Global Institute, 2021).

The bottom line is that the COVID-19 pandemic forced everyone to realize that much of what we once thought was impossible actually *was* possible—and we learned those lessons very quickly when the reality of the pandemic left us with no other options.

Armed with this knowledge, we now have a unique opportunity to guide our organizations out of this crisis by redesigning our workplace cultures, updating company policies, and eliminating outdated management practices and old ways of thinking about work that no longer fit. We will also need to significantly focus on our recruitment and retention strategies given that one in four employees are projected to quit once the pandemic ends (Mayer, 2021).

If we are successful in our efforts, we will not only make our workplaces more efficient, more effective, and more family-friendly, but we will also reduce otherwise significant expenditures through reductions in travel, less need for expensive office spaces, and reduced medical costs due to improved employee well-being. In addition, we will also reduce our collective environmental footprint due to less employee commuting to a specific office location and fewer business trips requiring air or car travel.

Though our current times are challenging, to be sure, they have also created an unparalleled opportunity for HR to play a starring role in their organizations. If we step up to proactively do what needs to be done to guide our organizations safely through these difficult times—and do it well—there will no longer be any doubt about the significance of HR's contribution to the organization. Instead, senior leaders will consistently *require* HR to be a part of critical business decisions going forward given the demonstrated and unquestionable value of their skills and insights to organizational success.

IMPLICATIONS FOR THE FUTURE

The COVID-19 pandemic has significantly impacted the nature of work and many of the changes are likely to re-shape the way we operate long after it is over (McKinsey Global Institute, 2021). Many of us are likely to continue to work remotely, to conduct our meetings via video conferencing, increase our use of document sharing tools, and continue to minimize our need to travel to conduct business—at least for the foreseeable future. As a result, organizations must rethink, reimagine, and reconsider how and where employees work in order to make the most of the post-pandemic reality.

Most of us have relied heavily on video conference calls during the pandemic. As a result, we have gotten to know one another a bit more personally given that more than a few of those calls have included unplanned sightings of children, pets, and an occasional spouse in the background. In other words, things got real. We cannot "un-see" what the pandemic revealed to us about the reality of the lives of our employees.

What that means is that employers can no longer ignore the fact that employees have both work and family/home responsibilities and that these duties sometimes collide. The reality is that children get sick, schools are sometimes closed for holidays that do not match up with the employer's schedule, the other parent may be required to travel for work, daycare sometimes closes (often without much notice) due to inclement weather, et cetera. To be clear, though, those issues did not begin with the pandemic—they just became significantly more visible.

In addition, the pandemic also exposed many vulnerabilities and cracks in our societal policies and institutional structures. We learned that when schools are not open to teach and care for our children, things quickly fall apart for employees. From working the front lines at higher rates to uneven gender roles giving them greater responsibilities at home, women have taken the brunt of the pandemic's impact (Gross, 2021; Kisner, 2021; Lewis, 2021; Lobell, 2021; "Women and the Pandemic," 2021).

With most schools and day cares closed, many employees have had to home-school and care for their children while working from home or they have had to change their hours to accommodate family demands, or both. As a result, countless families made the hard choice for at least one parent (usually the female) to leave their jobs during the past year and it is unclear whether they will return to the workforce after the pandemic ends (Haar, 2021; Lewis, 2021).

Organizational empathy and compassion toward the work-life struggles of employees seems to have increased over the past year due to a more holistic understanding of these tensions and conflicts that employees face on a daily basis. My hope is that it will spark employer action to proactively recruit and rehire many of the talented females who felt a need to leave their jobs during the pandemic. I am also hopeful that a majority of employers will voluntarily begin to offer family-friendly benefits, including flexible work schedules, opportunities to work remotely, childcare, and benefits that include childcare subsidies, among others.

Finally, we also learned that when millions of employees lose their jobs, they lose access to health insurance—a vital source of protection, especially during a major health crisis like a pandemic. It is all interconnected and it is a delicate balance. The pandemic has given us an unwelcome societal stress test, revealing the cracks and weaknesses in our institutions and our systems—and there are many. It laid bare the need for government and corporate policy initiatives that provide healthcare and childcare to support people and their families, both of which are essential for our society and for our organizations to effectively function.

The best employers will take whatever corporate actions that they can to support their employees while partnering with the U.S. government to put safeguards in place to address these larger societal issues. If policies and protections are enacted to address these significant work-family and healthcare issues, everyone wins—employees, their organizations, and our society at-large.

SPECULATION ABOUT OUR POSTPANDEMIC WORLD

Many academics and health experts have spent the past year issuing ominous warnings about the future; however, they have begun to shift their tone to "cautiously optimistic" now that vaccination rates are rapidly increasing in the United States (Hamblin, 2021). Still others continue to caution that the effects of the current pandemic are far from over and that we will be dealing with the risks and fear of this coronavirus for some time to come (Hixon, 2020; Huang, 2021).

The dismal consensus seems to be that the risk of future health crises of similar magnitude is almost guaranteed (Desmond-Hellman, 2020). Disruptive global health issues may indeed accelerate and become our new reality in the future. Whatever new crisis or challenge awaits us postpandemic, though, I have every confidence that HR practitioners—the organization's invisible heroes—will yet again rise to the occasion and meet that moment too.

AUTHOR'S NOTE

A heartfelt thanks to my colleague and friend, Dr Marilyn Faulkenburg, for her wise insights on an earlier draft of this chapter.

REFERENCES

Achor, S., Kellerman, G. R., Reece, A., & Robichaux, A. (2018, March 19). America's loneliest workers, according to research. *Harvard Business Review, 19.* https://hbr.org/2018/03/americas-loneliest-workers-according-to-research#:~:text=America's%20loneliest%20workers%20are%20single,heterosexual%2C%20and%20non%2Dreligious

Bingham, S. (2020, August 4). How HR leaders can adapt to uncertain times. *Harvard Business Review*. https://hbr.org/2020/08/how-hr-leaders-can-adapt-to-uncertain-times

Burrus, R. (2020), July 1). COVID-19 pandemic: Implications for managers and human resources. *Wilmington Biz Insights*. http://www.wilmingtonbiz.com/insights/robert__burrus/covid-19_pandemic_implications_for_managers_and_human_resources/2743

Campbell, M., & Gavett, G. (2021, February 10). What COVID-19 has done to our well-being, in 12 charts. *Harvard Business Review*. https://hbr.org/2021/02/what-covid-19-has-done-to-our-well-being-in-12-charts

Chawla, N., MacGowan, R. L, Gabriel, A. S., & Podsakoff, N. P. (2020). Unplugging or staying connected? Examining the nature, antecedents, and consequences of profiles of daily recovery experiences. *Journal of Applied Psychology, 105*(1), 19–39. https://doi.org/10.1037/apl0000423

Daniel, T. A. (2017, Winter). Managing toxic emotions at work: An examination of HR's unique role as the "organizational shock absorber." *Employment Relations Today, 43*(4), 13–19.

Daniel, T. A. (2018). *Managing toxic emotions at work: An empirical study of HR's role and its impact on personal well-being and organizational effectiveness*. https://doi.org/10.13140/RG.2.2.16315.26408

Daniel, T. A. (2020). *Organizational toxin handlers: The critical role of HR, OD, & coaching practitioners in managing toxic workplace situations*. Palgrave Macmillan.

Desmond-Hellmann, S. (2020, April 3). Preparing for the next pandemic. *Wall Street Journal*. https://www.wsj.com/articles/preparing-for-the-next-pandemic-11585936915

Devlin, J. (2021, March 9). How do you measure a year? *SHRM*. https://blog.shrm.org/blog/how-do-you-measure-a-year?utm_source=all&utm_medium=social&utm_campaign=communications~digital~how_do_you_measure_a_year?

Frost, P. J. (2003). *Toxic emotions at work*. Harvard Business School Press.

Frost, P. J. (2004). Handling toxic emotions: New challenges for leaders and their organizations. *Organizational Dynamics, 33*(2), 111–127.

Frost, P. J. (2006, March/April). Emotions in the workplace and the important role of toxin handlers. *Ivey Business Journal*. https://iveybusinessjournal.com/publication/emotions-in-the-workplace-and-the-important-role-of-toxin-handlers/

Grensing-Pophal, L. (2021, February 25). When hiring remotely raises legal issues. *SHRM-Talent Acquisition*. https://www.shrm.org/resourcesandtools/hr-topics/talent-acquisition/pages/when-hiring-remotely-raises-legal-issues.aspx

Gross, T. (2021, February 18). Almost a year into the pandemic, working moms feel "forgotten", journalist says. *NPR*. https://www.npr.org/2021/02/18/968930085/almost-a-year-into-the-pandemic-working-moms-feel-forgotten-journalist-says?utm_medium=social&utm_source=facebook.com&utm_term=nprnews&utm_campaign=npr

Haar, R. (2021, February 22). Women are leaving the workforce in droves. Here's what you should do before, during, and after a career break. *Time*. https://time.com/nextadvisor/in-the-news/women-in-the-workplace-career-break/?utm_source=facebook&utm_medium=social&utm_campaign=nextadvisor&utm_term=_&linkId=111893073

Hamblin, J. (2021, February 19). A quite possibly wonderful summer. *The Atlantic*. https://www.theatlantic.com/health/archive/2021/02/summer-2021-pandemic/618088/?utm_source=facebook&utm_campaign=the-atlantic&utm_term=2021-02-19T13%3A00%3A36&utm_content=edit-promo&utm_medium=social

Hixon, T. (2020, March 16). Get ready to live with COVID-19. *Forbes*. https://www.forbes.com/sites/toddhixon/2020/03/12/get-ready-to-live-with-covid-19.#26f55d347824

Huang, P. (2021, February 22). 'A Loss to The Whole Society': U.S. COVID-19 death toll reaches 500,000. *NPR*. https://www.npr.org/sections/health-shots/2021/02/22/969494791/a-loss-to-the-whole-society-u-s-covid-19-death-toll-reaches-500-000#:~:text=The%20Coronavirus%20Crisis-,'A%20Loss%20To%20The%20Whole%20Society'%3A%20U.S.%20COVID,19%20Death%20Toll%20Reaches%20500%2C000&text=via%20Getty%20Images-,On%20Jan.%2019%2C%20the%20incoming%20Biden%20administration%20hosted%20memorial%20to,another%20100%2C000%20Americans%20have%20died

Lewis, H. (2021, February 19). Listen: A disaster for women. *The Atlantic*. https://www.theatlantic.com/health/archive/2021/02/a-disaster-for-feminism/618096/?utm_content=edit-promo&utm_source=facebook&utm_medium=social&utm_term=2021-02-19T20%3A10%3A34&utm_campaign=the-atlantic

Lindzon, J. (2021, February 1). Why employers might not offer remote work options to junior staff. *Fast Company*. https://www.fastcompany.com/90596631/why-employers-might-not-offer-remote-work-options-to-junior-staff?utm_-source=facebook.com&utm_medium=social

Lobell, K. O. (2021, January 8). What HR professionals are looking forward to in 2021. *Society for Human Resource Management*. https://www.shrm.org/hr-today/news/hr-news/pages/what-hr-professionals-are-looking-forward-to-in-2021.aspx

Lumen, C. (September 15, 2020). Your HR manager is now your nurse, hall monitor, and remote IT liaison. *Fast Company*. https://www.fastcompany.com/90549764/your-hr-manager-is-now-your-nurse-hall-monitor-and-remote-it-liaison

Mayer, K. (2021, February 25). One in 4 workers plans to quit post-pandemic. *Human Resource Executive*. https://hrexecutive.com/one-in-4-workers-plans-to-quit-post-pandemic/?eml=20210301&oly_enc_id=4791B7303167C6Y

McKinsey Global Institute (2021, February). *The future of work after COVID-19*. https://www.mckinsey.com/featured-insights/future-of-work/the-future-of-work-after-covid-19

Mineo, L. (2021, February 18). Various innovations, rise of women leaders, greater collaboration between scientists, clinicians, to name a few. *The Harvard*

Gazette. https://news.harvard.edu/gazette/story/2021/02/finding-the-unexpected-positives-during-covid-times/

Nintex. (2021). *Nintex workplace 2021 study*. https://www.nintex.com/workplace-2021-study/

Prideaux, E. (2021, February 3). How to heal the "mass trauma" of Covid-19. *BBC Future*. https://www.bbc.com/future/article/20210203-after-the-covid-19-pandemic-how-will-we-heal

Segal, J. (2021, February 23). Updated OSHA and CDC guidance on #COVID-19 masks. *The SHRM Blog*. https://blog.shrm.org/blog/updated-osha-and-cdc-guidance-on-covid-19-masks?utm_source=all&utm_medium=social&utm_-campaign=communications~comms_general~updated_osha_and_cdc_guidance_on_%23covid-19_masks

Smith, A. (2021a, March 8). Take steps to fight pandemic fatigue. *SHRM*. https://www.shrm.org/ResourcesAndTools/legal-and-compliance/employment-law/Pages/coronavirus-fight-pandemic-fatigue.aspx

Smith, A. (2021b, February 25). CDC is depending on employers to encourage worker vaccinations. *SHRM*. https://www.shrm.org/ResourcesAndTools/legal-and-compliance/employment-law/Pages/coronavirus-CDC-encourage-worker-vaccinations.aspx

Society for Human Resource Management (n.d.). *Coronavirus and Covid-19 resources*. https://www.shrm.org/resourcesandtools/pages/communicable-diseases.aspx

U.S. Department of Labor. (2020). Families First Coronavirus Response Act. https://www.dol.gov/agencies/whd/pandemic/ffcra-employee-paid-leave

U.S. Department of the Treasury. (2020). Coronavirus Aid, Relief, and Economic Security (CARES) Act. https://home.treasury.gov/policy-issues/cares

U.S. Small Business Administration (2020–2021). Paycheck Protection Act. https://www.sba.gov/funding-programs/loans/coronavirus-relief-options/paycheck-protection-program

Women and the pandemic. (2021, March 3). *Time*. https://time.com/collection/women-covid19-pandemic/?utm_source=facebook&utm_medium=social&utm_campaign=women-and-the-pandemic&utm_term=_&linkId=112613016

World Health Organization. (2020, October 19). *Coronavirus disease (COVID-19)*. https://www.who.int/emergencies/diseases/novel-coronavirus-2019/question-and-answers-hub/q-a-detail/coronavirus-disease-covid-19

CHAPTER 2

SUPPLY CHAINS UNDER PANDEMIC PRESSURE

How to Build a More Resilient Supply Chain

Lathan Craig Austin

INTRODUCTION

Until the pandemic, supply chains largely went unnoticed by most individuals in the world economy, except for some business academics and supply chain professionals. While supply chains have often been acknowledged for their role in expanding trade and in improving commerce in recent decades, they have also endured substantial stresses upon their viability due to the effects of the recent pandemic, extreme weather events, and the simultaneously uneven rise of global trade. With such impacts more noticeable on the ability of supply chains to deliver to both businesses and individuals than in the past, there is now more public interest being directed at understanding how products can appear on a customer's doorstep or at least find themselves on a nearby business store's shelf. Indeed, with the onset of the COVID-19 pandemic in 2020, there is somewhat more recognition and even apprehension that well-performing supply chains are critical to our ability to control shortages and avoid

Back to a New Normal: In Search of Stability in an Era of Pandemic Disruption—Insight From Practitioners and Academics, pp. 15–24

delivery delays of both the mundane and the more essential products that transit within and across various industries (Page, 2020).

Supply chains within the global economy typically experience ever-shorter product life cycles, ever-shifting consumer tastes and wants, such that even small, unplanned disruptions within a supply chain can create rather unwelcome operational and financial results for an organization. Consider the beginnings of the pandemic when many could observe for themselves, could palpably feel, how this virus not only disrupted supply chains, but also fundamental aspects of their daily lives. Basic necessities, whether they were cleaning wipes, toilet paper, paper towels or various food items, became more difficult to locate, and in some cases, still remain scarce. This is evidence of supply chains seeking to adjust to new supplier and consumer-demand realities. This is an effort to seek a new delicate balance. Businesses are seeking to integrate the learning that the pandemic brought that altered their thinking on how to conduct business and how to manage their supply chains going forward. While the specific strategies may be diverse, they largely focus around on how to build better capabilities that ensure the organization is more resilient.

SEEING THE IMPACT OF THE PANDEMIC

While a number of firms were notably caught unprepared for the seismic shifts the pandemic brought to their supply chains, others were sufficiently nimble or agile enough to respond strategically to the ensuring changes that required rapidly repositioning their assets and resources so continued success could be assured. Many of the best practices adopted traditionally by management during prepandemic times still have relevance today and help create something of a blueprint for going forward. The emphasis on vetting multiple vendors for cost and reliability still continues. Businesses have traditionally chased efficiency, because they want to avoid the unnecessary cost of having their products just sit on the shelf while waiting for customers to purchase them.

At the same time, the role of supply chain organizations is not just about reducing or controlling costs. What the pandemic created and made clear was there is a shift in other emphases of supply chain management thinking. Where focus has always been on maintaining a lean inventory and pursuing a strategy of just-in-time production, this strategy always depended on there not being a "black swan" event occurring in the competitive environment, such as when China closed its economy in 2020, including its trade. When the pandemic struck, most organizations felt they possessed sufficiently robust continuity plans, but few found they had adequately planned for the utter scale of disruption that resulted.

Many businesses, however, relied on China for their manufacturing for everything from sophisticated gantry cranes to factory parts and dog food, so their supply chains were severely disrupted.

As the virus worked its way across the globe, more supply-chain chaos has ensued. Individuals that had been traditional office workers were now asked to stay at home, and many were uncertain how long this kind of corporate direction would last. As a result, many hoarded what they perceived as essentials, such as toilet paper and pasta, disturbing the natural equilibrium of a supply chain built on just-in-time deliveries that had always ensured that supermarket shelves stay stocked. Many automakers have witnessed their consumers just vanish away, while laptop manufacturers have struggled with great difficulty with just being able to build enough computers and monitors that could satiate the millions of people, who suddenly found they needed to connect via Zoom from home. These office workers had been transformed without much notice or planning into working from their homes, which had not been set up for that. This required looking at our homes in a new way, or at least, repurposing them.

LEARNING HOW TO RESPOND

Such events therefore necessitate a basic reorienting in business thinking on how to best manage supply chains during for all sorts of disruptive events, including pandemics. For supply chain managers, it is evident that a strategic view of organizational risk is currently underway that emphasizes the necessity of building up capabilities that allow business processes and assets to bounce back more quickly from potential logistics shocks, while still staying competitive. Many of these logistics events are largely predictable or can be anticipated, like the Suez Canal blockage, but resilience is essentially about benchmarking what others in the industry are doing so better capabilities for dealing with disruption can be constructed (Swink & Sanders, 2020).

Simultaneously, it is also about building strong relationships with supply chain partners so as to minimize product disruptions. Adopting just one supplier for obtaining ingredients for your products is unwise in most cases as it not always about cost or simplicity, but reliability in getting the necessary materials to use on time every time. Having strategic partners and one or two just-in-case firms that serve as backup is an essential strategy to pursue. The Suez Canal event is best framed as a common disruptive element to supply chains where the strategy among firms must be to plan for and minimize such events by making the organization more resilient by getting it better prepared for the next shocks that will certainly come to the supply chain. Some retail storefronts that shut down in early- to mid-2020 adapted their business models to allow them to turn their retail locations into distribution centers so as to meet demand.

Long-standing business continuity practices must be revisited so as to create stronger and more resourceful supply chains. It was clear during the pandemic that many companies with business continuity plans already constructed were nonetheless anxious for further improvement. This pandemic awakened them as a number of organizations saw that their business continuity planning provided little practical guidance to help the management team comprehend the multitude of interconnected effects that a black swan or random supply chain event creates. There are incredible breakthroughs in technology occurring that will change how goods and services move around the world for years to come. Inventory within these organizations cannot just be managed as a just-in-time orientation going forward, but it also must adopt a just-in-case framework for those black swan or even extreme weather events that always are in the pipeline. In the literature, such a strategy is framed as adopting resilience.

ADOPTING RESILIENCE

Resilience is therefore about supply chains and their members being able to recover from a logistics event and return to a normal state of doing business within a reasonable time frame of the episode (Mandal & Sarathy, 2018). It entails having the supply chain develop and possess a capacity to maintain operations even in the midst of a severe disruption. Indeed, there must exist something of a balance between the organization's capabilities it develops and maintains, and the vulnerabilities it faces. The winds of change always seem to blow in a competitive environment, but while it may not be possible for an organization to direct the wind, it is possible to raise sails in a business and adjust them, as may be needed from time to time.

As capabilities rise, potential vulnerabilities or weaknesses diminish. Clearly, disruption-oriented or disruption-prone organizations need to either construct capabilities that can reliably reconfigure the organization's resources or possess a risk-management resource management infrastructure that enables the realization of resilience. It has been found, however, that without being able to assess detailed information that suggests steps to be taken within an organization during a crisis, business continuity plans may be of little use for a firm. Analytics can be used to aid even more mature firms to employ digital playbooks that allow coordination of an organization's roles and responsibilities for its diverse people population across various functions. Much of the research on resilience though still remains mostly conceptual.

Given the many strategies a firm could develop, it is helpful to outline some priorities for creating a resilient supply chain. These include developing time-tested, reliable, and diverse networks of suppliers; being agile, whether it's regarding materials or logistics services, in responding to changing needs and situations; and employing sufficient technology to improve organizational decision-making and know what your supply chain is doing.

The pandemic witnessed how various manufacturers and retailers responded to the profound impact of this seismic event on their business environment by choosing to either limit the quantity of or reduce the variety of their product offerings. This was partly due to supplier constraints, changes in what consumers were buying, the inability of a key supplier to perform, and the typical logistics events in a given year, such as a plant fire, which is the most common event that affects supply chain activities. Such events can alter or destroy the well-being of an organization in terms of revenue loss or even increased costs if the firm's supply chain is not diversified enough where there is a stable of alternative vendors that have been vetted and can step into the breach when needed.

As intimated above, supply chains have evolved into exquisitely tuned machines that exude values such as efficiency and low costs. Traditionally, this allowed store shelves to remain full and customers to be assured that their products would likely be there. To ramp up production due to suddenly increased demand or carry larger inventories when consumers engage in panic buying cannot be factored in when forecasting a production. Larger inventories are anathema to for-profit corporations. If an organization carries more inventory due to its uncertainty that it will be able to order what it wants, the cost of this must show up in the products we buy. Similarly, government direction to get people to send their children back to school or encourage individuals to resume their past economic activities may seem logical for restarting the economy. It does not recognize, however, that consumers will not return unless they feel secure that the pandemic has been adequately addressed.

Thanks to the pandemic, consumers have become more aware that well-functioning supply chains matter for their continued well-being and in resolving shortages and delivery delays. Supply chains, however, need to adopt or at least embrace three priorities if they are to develop their capabilities of being more resilient to changes in their competitive environment (Uetz & Miller, 2020). Resiliency entails recovering from disruption and continuing business as usual, which depends on enlisting reliable suppliers, being extremely nimble with both organizational resources and logistics options, investing in technology, and developing capabilities that make visibility more likely.

PRIORITIES FOR REALIZING RESILIENCE

Develop a Supply Network That Is Built on Reliability, Trust, and Diversity

First, organizations within a supply chain orbit must construct a reliable, trusted, and diverse network of materials suppliers. This is not an activity that gets put together when your products or materials have just been disrupted. Resiliency is about anticipating disruption and preparing for it. There are many supply chain members, whether they be manufacturers or original equipment manufacturers, that benchmark themselves against what others across industries are doing, like Fiat Chrysler and Boeing, who are known to procure their parts and materials only from time-tested, quality-driven vendors across the globe. It is a world exhibiting complex risk for all who enter, so no individual business can be an island unto itself. High performers can coordinate with other partners in the supply chain by sharing the best practices available, by making sure each member's systems are strong enough to allow innovation across products, or by offering financial aid that ensures the survival of supply chain networks during disruptions.

The objective must always be to obtain reliable strategic sourcing that is attainable even during periods of intensely diverse supply chain disruptions, which can range themselves from extreme weather events, as in Texas, to a plant fire at a key vendor locale. Indeed, each event or activity within a supply chain enjoys some measure of inherent risk that an interruption to business will occur that results in unplanned costs of time, energy, and money to an organization. What is key here is that there is recognition that supply chains must be retooled in a manner that allows them to conduct operations even during these chance disruptive periods (Ivanov, 2020).

It is this extraordinary capacity to maintain continuity in business notwithstanding these unwelcome interruptions that embodies the true nature of resilience. It is a capability that is constructed by having trusted and varied vendors within an organization's working universe. Operational resilience rests on understanding that the supply chain must align its priorities with those of its suppliers.

Be Agile in Shifting Logistic Resources Around in Order to Both Respond to and Anticipate Changing Demand

Second, both in academia and in business, many are led to think that supply chains are nimble and flexible by nature, though most are not. As suggested above, for the last 3 decades, supply chain have been increasingly fine-tuned to achieve a high level of efficiency, which is a quite different kind of a value discipline than flexibility. Traditionally, most business management teams, or groups, have elected to pursue cost and efficiency as part of their strategy of keeping the firm profitable and its shareholders happy. More recently, supply chain managers have begun to rethink what it means to survive in today's competitive arena and have elected to also adopt robust risk mitigation strategies as part of ensuring the resiliency of their businesses.

Risk management or risk reduction entails having the supply chain and its constituents incorporate disruptive event readiness, construct a quick and effective response to an event, and restore the business back to its original state. The language that is most often used is agility or nimbleness, where manufacturers and shippers must be quick to answer so-called unexpected events or shifts in customer demand, because they should not be events that occur with much warning. It also entails the supply chain being able to bounce forward and adjust to a new normal. For example, the Retail Industry Leaders Association found that the quickness its retail supply chains were able to recover and answer the pandemic disruption on not just basic things like restocking and delivering goods to outlets or consumers directly, but also by its developed ability to maneuver and offer innovative offerings, such as curbside sales.

In addition to this restrategizing, what were traditionally transportation assets that were in house among most firms, have in recent years been outsourced to various third-party entities, whether they be UPS, FedEx, DHL, XPO, et cetera, which have themselves evolved to developing and offering logistics solutions for use by their clients. For these outsourcing organizations, it was a matter of both cost and a realization that owning transportation assets was no longer a core competency of the business and thus was outsourced. Amazon's strategy runs counter to this subcontracting trend and effort, given it elects to own its own transportation and logistics assets while it continues to be a very profitable retailer.

What is of critical importance is that the firm procure and enlist logistics providers that strategically add to the capabilities to make and fulfill the demand of either its clients or customers, which ensure a level of resiliency. And, as what is done with recruiting potential suppliers, choosing a reliable logistics carrier necessitates extreme vetting of the vendor's abilities to fit with the requirements of its organizational client. This suggests that these third-party logistics entities have suitable enough technology that makes possible not only the tracking of individual shipments, but also collects actionable and timely information that ensures better decision-making and planning can occur that advances the strategic interests of the firm.

Make Technology Serve as a Transforming Tool

Third, e-commerce and the adoption of resiliency have become intertwined within firms. The pandemic has simply accelerated trends and planning already underway, such as placing more business transactions online simultaneously with digitizing information so critical for improving decision-making on the corporate level. Artificial intelligence and machine learning enable organizations of all sizes to digest enormous amounts of data to create actionable data. This allows better collaboration, negotiation, and problem-solving, such that various scenarios can be run that predict the most likely outcomes, which then suggest options for managers, based on the organization's objectives. Such technology greatly aids supply chain visibility and agility thanks to better risk management (Association for Supply Chain Management, 2021).

Artificial intelligence-powered machine vision inspections, for example, similar to those employed by both Amazon and DHL, enable the organizations to reduce error rates and expedite trailer unloading to just thirty minutes. Similarly, robotic process automation allows tasks such as billing, invoicing, production planning, and even carrier selection. Artificial intelligence technologies can also make easier the sophisticated and laborious process of constructing and keeping up digital playbooks that help guide groups across various organizational functions with the best recommended course of action to pursue.

Resilient organizations must employ software and digitization so as to assess accurately their internal operations. Digital technology must be mirrored across the entire supply chain, including vendors, manufacturers, retailers, and logistics carriers. Reaping such valuable information gleaned from technology-based transparency enables firms to increase their knowledge of what their business is doing at any one moment, which supports the development of resiliency. It is crucial that your system be able to talk to the systems of your supply chain members, which means that you are sharing data. Given the reticence of shippers to replace or update their logistics systems infrastructure, logistics management software is regrettably not tightly integrated as it needs to be, given its broad products suites, such that it limits widespread or improved functionality.

Construct capabilities that ensure real-time visibility through more intense use of technologies and collaborative processes to meet customer's expectations and limit the bullwhip effect.

The bullwhip effect refers to a possible inaccurate demand forecasting, due to order amplification that can result in added supply chain costs; bullwhip effect causes inventory levels to rise artificially due to sudden demand as in a panic. Such unplanned costs include shortage and back-order costs.

The competitive marketplace is currently enjoying an enormous wave of digitization and even accelerated innovation that is helped by large amounts of investment from various sources of private money and venture capital. What this digitation does is greatly aid visibility in terms all parties in a supply can see the status of their shipment, which is a development that makes possible being able to calculate demand while also improving the customer experience. Having digital and automated technology does not by itself enable resiliency within an organization, but it does initiate the necessary first step. Visibility begins to realize its strategic value when it enables or increases the organization's ability to reconfigure itself as needed to meet its competitive threats or market opportunities.

Visibility is not itself recognized universally as a logistics capability that a firm can construct. It may better be construed as a strategic goal that an organization aspires. Visibility must enable the organization or its supply chain to develop logistics capabilities, whether they be a robust technology, internal and interorganizational collaborative processes, or the adoption of resiliency to potential disruptions that can upend the ability of the organization to enjoy continued success.

Visibility best prepares the firm and its supply chain members to share better the accessibility and sharing of information. Such information is strategically employed to adjust production plans to reflect changing demand, to update the delivery schedule of shipments, and permits a firm to carry leaner inventories that allow the reducing of costs and the reduction of the bullwhip effect.

This suggests that supply chains can then be more market responsive and quicker to weather disruptions to the transit of their products and materials if they have access to the information that allows them to respond and act timelier. Logistics capabilities, which include resiliency, permit the firm to augment its resiliency by ensuring information sharing is readily shared and of higher quality across the supply chains, thus allowing visibility, such that improved decision-making can be made timelier and accurately that shows up on the bottom line. Often, the view of supply chains for many firms is based simply on the available internal data, or relies on a siloed unit's outlook, or does not represent current data. This greatly limits the organization's ability to discover emerging threats or ascertain how much a disruption may impact across various supply chains and business units.

Lastly, the pandemic has shown that organizations must improve and prioritize their integration with fellow supply chain partners. For example, the pharmaceutical sector has struggled to integrate with suppliers through a better exchange of data. What had become clear during much of 2020 was that supply chain members were not using the same interface or even the same system so gathering information was laborious in terms of collecting and analyzing. Improving visibility therefore demands the various organizations to embrace data governance, data exchange protocols, and categorization, end to end, across the supply chain; otherwise, both visibility and its sister, resiliency, are seriously impaired.

REFERENCES

Association for Supply Chain Management. (2021). *The resilient supply chain benchmark: Ready for anything? Turbulence and the resilience imperative.* ASCM. https://www.ascm.org/eiu-benchmark/

Ivanov, D. (2020). Viable supply chain model: Integrating agility, resilience and sustainability perspectives—Lessons from and thinking beyond the COVID-19 pandemic. *Annals of Operations Research,* 1–21. https://doi.org/10.1007/s10479-020-03640-6

Mandal, S., & Sarathy, R. (2018). The effect of supply chain relationships on resilience: Empirical evidence from India. *Global Business Review, 19*(6), 196–217. https://doi.org/10.1177/0972150918758094

Page, P. (2020, June 5). Today's logistics report: Hobbled factory supply chains; trade flows sliding; hedging for recovery. *The Wall Street Journal.* https://www.wsj.com/articles/todays-logistics-report-hobbled-factory-supply-chains-trade-flows-sliding-hedging-for-recovery-11591366825?mod=searchresults&page=1&pos=3

Swink, M., & Sanders, N. (2020, November 9). Want to build a supply chain? Focus on capabilities. *Supply Chain Management Review, 24*(6), 12–21. https://www.scmr.com/article/want_to_build_a_digital_supply_chain_focus_on_capabilities

Uetz, A., & Miller, V. (2020, November 2). Supply chain strategy trends: COVID-19 is prompting executives to reconsider resilience. *Supply Chain Management Review.* https://www.scmr.com/article/supply_chain_strategy_trends_covid_19_is_prompting_executives_to_reconsider?utm_source=TWISC&utm_medium=NLT

CHAPTER 3

HEALTHCARE AND THE COVID-19 PANDEMIC

Caring for Those Who Care for Us

Rebecca D. Carpenter

The effects of the COVID-19 pandemic permeated itself globally manifesting itself in the initiation of various forms of response. Governments initiated unprecedented public health interventions, such as, lockdowns, widespread viral testing, the mandating of the wearing of masks, and social distancing, as efforts to control the viral spread. Unfortunately, some of these initiated efforts began after the virus had affected a significant portion of the population and began to infiltrate into other countries. This rapid viral spread resulted in a significant health and social crisis affecting the economic sustainability of many countries, creating conflicts and competition over scarce resources.

The ongoing pandemic intensified fears of a global economic crisis and potential recession. Reductions in workforce availability resulted from social distancing requirements, required self-isolation post exposure, force lockdowns, and restricted travel, across all socioeconomic sectors resulting in many lost opportunities for employment. However, the demand for medical supplies significantly increased as the volume of

Back to a New Normal: In Search of Stability in an Era of Pandemic Disruption—Insight From Practitioners and Academics, pp. 25–43

patients treated by frontline healthcare professionals (FHP) for the COVID-19 virus surged (Nicola et al., 2020).

The requirements facing FHP as they cared for the increasing number of patients, and the unfortunate percentage of deaths associated with the virus, took a toll on the mental and physical health of these individuals. Without consideration of the need to address the concerns experienced by these professionals, the potential for long-term effects significantly increased. FHP experienced emotional exhaustion and job burnout as they attempted to cope with the patient care aspects associated with the provision of care for individuals with COVID-19. The unpreparedness and the unknowns associated with the virus increased the likelihood of a negative outcome would result in regard to the mental and physical health of these essential professionals as stress, exhaustion and the potential for viral contraction themselves rose to critical levels.

In addition, this unprecedented, nonprepared COVID-19 global pandemic created moral dilemmas and conflicts for healthcare professionals resulting from the virus' rapid spread, outpacing available resources, thus creating inconsistent, noncoordinated decisions in regard to the provision and allocation of patient care and resources. This chapter examines one aspect of the pandemic response, the distribution and management of resources during the COVID-19 pandemic from the perspective of the FHP and the development of subsequent recommendations for postpandemic outcomes and future events.

SETTING THE STAGE

Conflict quickly arose for those individuals involved in providing frontline care to patients with COVID-19. The source of this conflict evolved from multiple avenues. First, being an FHP meant firsthand exposure with an increased risk for contracting the virus. This fear of contracting the virus, in addition to concern for the possible exposure of family members, increased the stress normally associated with healthcare. In addition, the scarcity of personal protective equipment (PPE) and the greater risk of complications for older healthcare professionals and those with underlying medical conditions compounded the stress thus facilitating the likelihood of potential conflicts.

For FHP, there exists a duty to provide care. This obligation includes knowingly exposing themselves to known and unknown risks. However, FHP also have duties to themselves and others beyond the patients they serve. Each additional role a healthcare professional has, that is, spouse, father, mother, parent, et cetera, has ascribed to it certain obligations. When dealing with a pandemic, these roles can go unfulfilled thus creating additional sources of stress and anxiety. Their obligation to the care of their patients can create conflict with their duties to others. In comparison to other major events such as the aftermath of mass shooting, bombing, or weather-related injuries, where required care provided amounts to hours or days, care during this pandemic labored on for weeks, then months and over a year. This altered time frame of care provision increased stress levels and contributed to the potential for conflict, internal and external.

FHP faced challenges and encountered situations they had not previously confronted during their training and in their careers. The unknowns significantly contributed to the fear and anxiety experienced by frontline healthcare professionals. This was a complicated problem with responsibilities for minimizing risks requiring collaborative efforts of the hospitals, the healthcare system, the government, and the healthcare professionals. Therefore, management decisions should be collaborative and transparent to reduce potential conflict and promote ethical behavior.

The core concepts of ethical principles include beneficence, justice, autonomy, and nonmaleficence. These principles are fundamental in the patient-healthcare professional relationship (Rawlings et al., 2020). However, although these principles remain consistent, the application of these principles may change based on the circumstances encountered, especially during a time of crisis like the COVID-19 pandemic. Beneficence involves actions directed toward the best interest of others and the avocation of another's well-being. Justice involves the treating of individuals fairly, being impartial and reasonable. Autonomy involves making your own choices, determining your best interest. Finally, Nonmaleficence means not harming anyone or the taking of actions to avoid harm. While these ethical principles remained during the pandemic, their application changed resulting in interpersonal conflicts for FHP.

INTERPERSONAL TURMOIL

Interpersonal conflict stems from incompatibilities, differences or disagreements between individuals. In this case, interpersonal conflict arose in those FHP involved in providing direct care to patients with COVID-19. Responses to this conflict took on differing forms. Some professionals responded by standing up for their rights as well as the rights of their patients (competing). Others reacted by putting their patents before the safety of themselves (accommodating). Additionally, others refused to acknowledge or deal with the conflict (avoiding). As a healthcare professional, they also attempted to work with others to resolve the conflict (collaboration). Alternatively, professionals tried to develop a solution benefiting all those involved (compromising). In looking at the situation, which occurred during this pandemic, FHP often exhibited more than one of these coping mechanisms as they pushed through the conflicts associated with and arising from situations created by the pandemic.

However, many situations in healthcare are not black or white. Those "gray" areas contributed to the conflict felt by FHP during this pandemic. The challenges encountered during the response to this pandemic such as, the rapid spread of the virus, the large number of acutely ill patients, the associated loss of life, the scarcity of PPE, the limited capacity of intensive care unit beds, and ventilators left the healthcare industry with the problem of ethically managing resources. This continual pressure and stress sent interpersonal conflicts on a downward spiral.

The change in the delivery of healthcare resulting from the COVID-19 pandemic altered the focus of patient care from the individual patient to the overall well-being of many patients. During a pandemic situation, the equitable distribution determination of available resources involves situations not routinely considered in an environment of adequate resources. This includes the limited availability of frontline healthcare professionals themselves who have altered their practices to caring for an increasing number of patients with limited resources.

EXAMINING THE ISSUE

The COVID-19 pandemic resulted in the shortage of many healthcare related resources including medical supplies. As the virus rapidly spread globally, depleting available medical supplies, the result was ongoing negotiations/bidding to obtain needed resources. As the virus continued to surge, countries began to restrict exporting of medical supplies. This resulted in an imbalance in the distribution of supplies along the medical supply chain. Countries like the United States, as well as other more technologically advanced countries, curtailed the exporting of medical equipment such as ventilators. However, China and other Western Asian countries were the primary manufacturers of masks, medical gowns and surgical gloves (PPE), which soon became scarce in the United States as these countries curtailed exports of these items to meet their internal needs.

As a result, countries and individual U.S. states entered a negotiation/bidding battle to obtain available resources. This negotiation/bidding for medical supplies during the pandemic has focused attention on the existing supply chain for medical resources especially PPE and the policy implications surrounding their manufacture and distribution. The rapid spread of the COVID-19 virus shutdown the world's major economies causing havoc on global trade and medical supply distribution. Although it is unrealistic for any one country to produce all the medical supplies needed efficiently in the event of a pandemic, growing is a national concern related to the quick and rapid depletion and subsequent unavailability of medical supplies.

The issue in regard to the availability of needed medical supplies stems from the perspective upon which the global supply chain for PPE is considered. Although healthcare organizations view the acquisition and storage of medical supplies from a "just-in-time" perspective, to reduce overhead costs and potential expiration of products, this perspective creates an unstable, fragile supply chain when a crisis ensues. One way to prevent this shortage from occurring postpandemic is for healthcare organizations to have a robust and enlarged storage capacity and process for rotation of supplies to prevent expiration and to assess for additional sources for supplies rather than a reliance on only one supply source. This is accomplished through: enlargement of the storage capacity for medical supplies; expansion of the number of international and domestic production sites to reduce dependency on a single source supply chain; identification of growing end markets that can join in an international production network; and fostering the development of domestic production and research and development with related industries (Gereffi, 2020).

United States companies have continued to locate production of goods offshore. This practice, while reducing the overhead costs associated with the manufacture and distribution of products, enhancing the economies of scale, providing greater flexibility, increasing access to low cost labor, and improving distribution logistics, has the negative potential to breakdown during a crisis. The global medical supply industry has its own unique governance structure, which can affect coordination of product along the supply chain. Each component of the medical supply chain is specialized so if there is a disruption in one component along the chain it affects those entities upstream and downstream. During the COVID-19 pandemic, the differences in the manufacturing time frame for medical supplies was due to differing global lockdowns disrupting the process along various points in the supply chain. In addition, the varying conditions and needs in each country contributed to the scarcity of medical supplies (Gereffi, 2020).

In a globally dependent medical supply chain, the value of the components is unevenly distributed. Some parts of the manufacturing process are specialized requiring greater skill and knowledge, and often additional time to complete. All these factors, while during noncrisis periods work efficiently; during a global crisis have the potential to breakdown creating devastating effects downstream. In addition, during the COVID-19 pandemic, countries exerted export controls restricting the flow of medical supplies, thus compounding the shortage (Gereffi, 2020). This is what occurred during the early stages of this pandemic.

The increase in demand for medical supplies, due to the rapid spread of the virus, created an expanded international demand. The diversity of the manufacture of medical supplies, the reliance on an expansive, but often single source supply chain, and the difficulty controlling and regulating the production flow during the pandemic contributed to the medical supply shortage. Below is a 2018 list of the top exporters of medical supplies required to care for patients safely and effectively during the COVID-19 pandemic:

- textile face mask: China 50.4%; Germany 6.3%; United States 5.3%;
- protective garments: China 42.8%; Cambodia 6.6%; Belgium 5.6%;
- surgical gloves: Malaysia 39.1%; Thailand 20.1%; China 9.7%;
- protective goggles: China 48%; United States 6.1%; Germany 5.7%;
- masks with mechanical parts: Germany 19.6%; United Kingdom 16.8%; United States 16.2%;
- other gloves: Malaysia 59.3%; Thailand 14.1%; China 8.4%;
- paper bed sheets: China 23.9%; Germany 8.2%; United States 7.5%;
- needles, catheters and cannulae: United States 19.6%; Ireland 13%; Mexico 11.3%;
- intubation kits: United States 17.7%; Germany 14.1%; Mexico 11.9%; and
- patient monitoring devices: United States 22%; Japan 14.4%; Germany 12% (Gereffi, 2020, pp. 290–291).

Examining the location and percentage of product production of exporters of medical supplies, used for caring for patients with the COVID-19 virus, provides visual representation of how the restrictions on exports and the varying degrees of country lockdowns contributed to the shortage of medical supplies.

According to these 2018 statistics, the top exporters of medical supplies needed for the caring of patients during the COVID-19 pandemic (accounting for 50% of the trade) included Germany (15%); the United States (11%); Switzerland (9%); China (8%); and Ireland (8%). In regard to imports, the United States had 18% of the imports of medical supplies needed for the COVID-19 pandemic, with Germany second at 9%. The

United States and Germany tend to specialize in those higher technological items (that is, ventilators), while China and Malaysia specialize in those bedside medical supplies healthcare professionals need to protect themselves and to care for their patients. This breakdown indicates the interdependencies between medical supply manufacture and distribution created an asymmetrical relationship (Gereffi, 2020, pp. 290–291).

An example of this are the face masks, an essential component to help reduce the spread of a primarily airborne virus. Under nonpandemic conditions, face masks are a relatively cheap commodity to manufacture. However, there are specific guidelines for the higher specialty masks, the N95. Although the manufacturing of surgical masks and N95 face masks are similar, the filtering components for the N95 face masks have additional steps in the manufacturing process requiring extra time and costs. At the beginning of the pandemic, China was the main producer of surgical masks. However, being at the center of the viral outbreak, China did not have the face mask capacity to meet its own needs, thus curtailing the amount available for export. This left the United States and other countries who relied on the importing of face masks from China in a dilemma. In addition, the United States faced internal strife, as those U.S. manufacturers of the N95 face masks could not meet the demand of U.S. healthcare professionals due to their export commitments to other countries.

The invoking of the Defense Production Act of 1950 began to help this dilemma; however, its enactment caused an upheaval within the U.S. manufacturers and some of our allies. Manufacturers were upset because their ability to export was restricted, and allies were upset because those that relied on the U.S. manufacturers for their face mask supplies were cutoff. This required U.S. manufacturers to attempt to increase production amidst our own lockdowns and a reduced available workforce. However, the desire to produce additional face masks created openings for new entrants into the market. It also required ongoing negotiations/bidding to acquire the supplies needed by healthcare professionals (Gereffi, 2020).

Finally, the just-in-time model for medical supplies in the United States left the country vulnerable. This model promotes lean production on the part of medical supply manufacturers, and low inventories for healthcare facilities. This model resulted in the unwavering expansion of global manufacturing of medical supplies. Less inventory on hand affords an opportunity for manufacturers to increase their cash flow and operating margins, thus remaining more competitive. While this makes sense during "normal" periods, it left the healthcare industry and the country vulnerable during this crisis as witnessed during the COVID-19 pandemic (Gereffi, 2020).

Although the just-in-time model helps reduce associated costs and reduced inventories, it creates an unstable supply chain in the event of a crisis. Supply chains for needed medical supplies have not been expanding globally, and countries have become increasingly dependent on exports from certain economies such as China and other Asian countries. To prevent what transpired during the COVID-19 pandemic from occurring again in regard to the availability of medical supplies, and to establish a more crisis-resilient supply chain, the United States needs to look at ramping up production of these required medical supplies within its own borders. This reduces the dependency on other countries to supply needed equipment in the event of a future pandemic. This also allows for new entrants into the market creating competition and lowering costs (Gereffi, 2020).

Another protection against what occurred during this pandemic is to increase global manufacturing sites so required supplies are not dependent upon one or two manufacturing locations. This will result in expanded end markets benefiting an international network. Finally, priority should be to foster innovation through the promotion of research and development and collaboration with companies in related industries. Diversification of the risk is essential to prevent a reoccurrence of the medical supply shortfalls encountered during the COVID-19 pandemic. While offshore manufacturing will continue to be a major component in the medical supply chain, the development of regional supply chains would reduce the risk faced during a crisis. China remains a significant competitor both for the manufacturing of medical supplies and as a market for U.S. medical exports. Local partnerships between public-private entities, which occurred during the pandemic, need continuing to help prevent a repeat of the shortages in the event of a future pandemic. (Gereffi, 2020).

The COVID-19 pandemic exposed deficiencies in preparedness, policies and global supply chain adequacy. Trying to secure needed medical supplies, resulted in numerous negotiations/bidding as countries tried to take care of the expanding viral spread within their borders, conserve their internal supplies of scarce medical supplies and equipment, and compete globally for available resources. Responses during the COVID-19 pandemic revealed a fragmented medical supply chain with manufacturing of essential supplies occurring in only one or two primary locations. This weakness, in combination of a just-in-time model for the healthcare industry in regard to manufacture and storage of medical supplies, provided the ingredients for an uncoordinated, inadequate initial response to the pandemic. Recovery took time and continued as a second surge began shortly after the Thanksgiving and Christmas holidays in 2020. Needed is a close and honest evaluation of the medical supply chain and the negotiations/bidding involved in these processes. Without this evaluation, there is no accountability for mistakes made and allowances made to incorporate the knowledge gained, thus creating a vulnerability and risk an inadequate response would occur again in the future.

In addition, there needs to be an increased transparency into the manufacture and distribution of medical supplies. The behind the scenes negotiations and subcontracting created a vulnerability and a risk for the healthcare industry, which came to the surface during the COVID-19 pandemic. Arising from the medical supply scarcity brought on by the pandemic is a concern supplies will be substandard with quality compromised in an attempt to meet demand. Consideration of this risk requires the institution of safeguards to insure supplies meet required standards. There also needs to be contingency plans in place should medical supply chains breakdown as they did during this pandemic. The just-in-time model may not be the best course of action for the healthcare industry to mitigate future risks in regard to medical supplies. In addition, the reliance on only one or two medical supply manufacturers in a global pandemic carries the associated risk of inadequate supplies as witnessed during the COVID-19 pandemic.

The importance is to examine the lessons learned and apply it to knowledge from the past to be better prepared in the future. In additional to the adequate availability of medical supplies and the identified need to reevaluate the medical supply chain, rising to the top of are additional needs to sustain the healthcare industry during the time of a pandemic: defined resource allocation, transparency and trust, and effective communication.

DEFINED RESOURCE ALLOCATION

Unfortunately, the effects on societal behavior and the delivery of healthcare changed drastically during the COVID-19 pandemic. The result was the need to provide care for disease and critical conditions outpaced the available resources designed to care for these illnesses. Having to allocate and function within a scarce resource environment is not something familiar to most FHP, especially here in the United States. Therefore because of the intensity and sensitivity of the pandemic environment, when the situation presents itself, the burden of any resource allocation decision should reside with a team rather than solely dependent on the FHP (Rawlings et al., 2020).

An ethics framework for the distribution of scarce resources during a pandemic should be designed to help those FHP, hospital leadership and policymakers determine how best to distribute and manage available resources. However, the framework should not be the definitive end to the issue, but rather be a basis upon which to consider those particular circumstances present. The ideal framework would provide guiding questions to ask in making the decision (Dawson et al., 2020).

In addition, the framework should balance the duty of care promoting equality and equitable distributions of associated risks and societal benefits (McCullough, 2020). FHP are individual patient-focused and the shift to care guided by considerations for public health and societal concerns creates stress, anxiety and tension for those professionals. This was especially true with the COVID-19 pandemic where many FHP had never experienced anything like this or trained in emergency procedures with scarce resources. Finally, the recommendation is those involved in making the decisions should represent diverse communities for the inclusion of cultural differences since the virus affects racial and ethnic groups differently (Schoch-Spana et al., 2020).

Whenever resources are scarce and unable to meet the need or the demand, decisions made determine the allocation of resources and require ethical considerations. Decisions should be consistent and thought out. However, decisions made relating to the scarce availability of resources will be controversial. If a decision making process is consistent and agreed on by all parties involved, the decisions have a greater chance of acceptance even if not all parties involved agree. Characteristics of a resource allocation decision process would be one that is transparent, include the reasons for the decision, who made the decision, and if there can be a revision in the decision should new evidence present. Although in reality this may not always be possible due to the time constraints on the decision, this should be the foundation for resource allocation (Dawson et al., 2020).

Emanuel et al. (2020) outlined four ethical values and principles to direct the distribution of scarce resources during a pandemic. These include the maximizing of benefits (save the most lives /life-years), the treatment of individuals equally (first-come first served, random selection), the encouragement and rewarding of value (retrospective, individuals who have made relevant contributions/ prospective, individuals who are likely to contribute), and the giving to those in worst condition (sickest/youngest; Emanuel et al., 2020, p. 2052). However, FHP do not like being in the position of making those decisions. Their training is to care for all patients to the best of their ability.

Dawson et al. (2020) suggested characteristics of a resource allocation decision include an equal value for all involved; priority to those activities enabling getting the most out of available resources; and the giving priority to those in the greatest need. The overall goal is to get the most value from the use of the resource. However, determining the "most value" will differ depending on the situation and circumstances. The responsibility of FHP is to do what is best for their patients. This continues during a pandemic. However, methods for carrying this out differs. For example, patients cannot have visitors due to the ability of the virus to spread. Being able to visit and to have visitors is the norm during nonpandemic periods. This contributes to stress and fear for patients, families and healthcare professionals (Dawson, et al., 2020). The importance here is have a foundational plan for the allocation of scarce resources. Having transparent and ongoing communication between all parties involved develops trust and reduces the degree of stress, anxiety and fear associated with clinical process restrictions.

TRANSPARENCY AND TRUST

Transparency and trust, is the path healthcare organizational leaders should follow during and postpandemic. The path healthcare leaders choose to follow, and the behavior exhibited will influence the outcomes during as well as postpandemic. During times of crisis requires a transformational leader who makes sense out of the situation for his/her employees, promotes the use of technology to its fullest capacity, provides for their employee's safety and well-being; and is an innovative and transparent communicator; all while sustaining the business or organization (Dirani et al., 2020, p. 340).

This has been a challenge for healthcare leaders as they try and maintain a positive bottom line, meet their patients' needs, while carefully considering the safety of their employees and the organization. With change occurring each day during a pandemic, with the ebb and flow of the level and degree of viral spread, and the ever-changing guidelines and restrictions imposed, this is difficult. Some healthcare leaders successfully sustained their organizations during the pandemic, while others did not. Faced with unprecedented challenges, healthcare leaders have found themselves struggling to sustain their bottom lines. This is true for the healthcare organizations whose leaders found themselves lacking in available resources and unprepared for the magnitude of the pandemic. These real threats to the safety of both patients and staff made the ethical distribution of scarce resources more difficult to manage.

Faced with unprecedented challenges related to the COVID-19 pandemic, leaders within the healthcare industry had to make decisions based on their personal instincts and knowledge. Having never experienced these challenges before, the outcomes of these decisions varied among organizations. Some healthcare leaders successfully navigated through this uncharted period, while others unfortunately failed. There is a distinction between leadership behaviors needed during noncrisis times and those needed during crisis times. Those leaders exhibiting "crisis" needed behaviors are successful in pushing ahead during a pandemic (Dirani et al, 2020, p. 340).

According to (Dirani et al., 2020, p. 340), "leadership practices" that are displayed during noncrisis times need to shift to "leadership roles" during a crisis. The leadership practices indicate during a noncrisis period leaders should, "model the way; inspire a shared vision; challenge the process; enable others to act; and encourage the heart (Dirani, et al, 2020, 340). In comparison, the leadership roles propose that during a crisis period leaders should, "be a sensemaker; be a technology enabler; promote emotional stability and employee well-being; be an innovative communicator; and maintain the financial health of the organization" (Dirani et al., 2020, p. 340).

As organizations strive to maintain sustainability during a pandemic, the role of healthcare organizational leadership becomes increasingly important. As observed during the pandemic, many organizations were unable to continue operation resulting from the inability to maintain financial health. They were unable to shift previous processes to new ways of remaining connected to their customer base. This was no different in regard to FHP who looked toward their leaders for guidance and information. Those leaders able to adjust their approach and guide their organizations through this crisis will have a stronger team on the other side.

According to (Dirani et al., 2020, p. 334), leadership needs realigned to exhibit the following four skills. First, healthcare leaders must be display "positive accountability." This requires a healthcare leader to be able to recognize and identify how their employees individually manage stress. Some healthcare organizations have taken a "holistic" response to meet employees' needs by taking into consideration employees' mental, emotional and physical needs. Second, healthcare leaders need to tune into communication within the organization to address and stop misinformation. Healthcare leaders need to be transparent and keep the channel of communication flowing in both directions. In addition, monitoring of the environment to identify issues/conflicts when they arise must occur by healthcare leaders, addressing them immediately before they escalate (Dirani et al., 2020, p. 334).

Third, healthcare leaders need to place their employees above themselves. Their focus should be on employees' needs and meeting these needs. Healthcare leaders should reinforce their gratitude for the efforts put forth by their employees. Finally, healthcare leaders need to be flexible and adapt quickly. With personal feelings placed aside, information needs to be processed and quickly disseminated, needs and activities need prioritization, and finally healthcare leaders should resist the tendency for impulsive reactions (Dirani et al., 2020, p. 334).

Healthcare leaders cannot afford to lose their skilled workforce if they want to continue to meet customer and business needs. Healthcare leaders should focus attention and efforts on their employees acknowledging that individuals react differently to stress, conflict and crisis and should continually develop avenues to connect with all employees to help them navigate through these unsettling times. A crisis sends fear and uncertainty through any workforce. Disruptions becomes the norm rather than the exception. Healthcare leaders should provide their employees a variety of solutions to sustain them through this pandemic. Needed are innovative and creative ideas to meet the needs of frontline healthcare professionals. FHP want and need reassurance and the ability to balance work/life, which has taken on new identities during this pandemic.

EFFECTIVE COMMUNICATION

Communication, although challenging during a crisis, is the important element in the management of stress during a crisis. During a crisis, communication from healthcare leaders should be transparent, contain the information employees need, and want to know, as well as reviewing what they already know. Communications should also contain information about services that are available to help them cope with emotional and mental health concerns; and continually acknowledge how difficult the situation is for their employees, and how much their efforts are appreciated (Dirani, et al., 2020, p. 334).

Effective communication is the essential element-helping healthcare organizations navigate through rapid changes. It is through organizational communications that employees are able to process, understand, manage, and cope with change. Without ongoing and continual communication, employee fear, anxiety and stress increases, leading to conflicts. A high level of uncertainty will manifest itself in reduced or poor performance having negative consequences for the organization and the employees. Without effective and ongoing communication through periods of change, employees may develop feelings of resentment, resist changes the organization is attempting to implement, and disengage from organizational attempts to change (Li et al., 2021).

Transparent communication, during a time of a pandemic, could positively affect the ability of employees to cope with change and improve the relationship between the organization and their employees, reducing the potential for conflicts. The COVID-19 pandemic was an event, which quickly rose to a crisis level for healthcare organizations. The challenges that were encountered arose rapidly requiring healthcare organizations and FHP to react quickly often without time to plan the response. There were so many unknowns associated with the virus that healthcare organizations frequently adjusted their responses to protect their employees, sustain the organization, and meet patient needs. There was often not much time to plan a response. The performance of planning, simultaneously as changes were implemented, further contributed to employee anxiety, stress and negatively affecting their ability to cope with and manage the changes and any conflicts that arose.

When employees face sudden, unplanned change, they have a need for information about organizational expectations. Li et al. (2021) found employee participation in organizational decision-making, the receipt of ongoing information and transparent communication provides employees with the tools needed to cope with and manage change. Based upon the information provided to them, employees process the information forming the foundation upon which they derive mechanisms for coping and managing the changes, they are encountering. In contrast to just providing information, when organizations provide transparent and consistent communication to their employees, and take accountability for performing these actions, employees are better equipped with the resources they need for proactive coping with changes in the work environment. This detailed form of communication not only conveys information, but it also provides employees with the rationale upon which the organization made the decision. If employees have a role in making the decisions, they feel like they are a part of the process for arriving at a solution.

In addition, Li et al. (2021) anticipated that the use of transparent communication would have long-term positive effects on employee/organizational relationships postpandemic. The implementation and ongoing use of transparent communication not only helps employees navigate through the changes imposed in response to the pandemic, but it will also strengthen the connection between employees and their organizations. The postpandemic environment is something healthcare organizations need to consider as they develop responses to situations encountered. Communication in general can create many challenges. However, during a time of crisis, such as the COVID-19 pandemic, these challenges intensify. Unfortunately, during a pandemic, these communications continue to evolve so the goal becomes to balance the information with the avoidance of panic and increased anxiety. Founded upon the concept of doing no harm to others and respecting individual rights and privacy, communication should be honest, sincere and comprehensible, and supply the needed information that is, the status of medical supplies (Guttman & Lev, 2020).

SUSTAINING FRONTLINE HEALTHCARE PROFESSIONALS

FHP especially those in intensive care units (ICUs) experience large amounts of stress and pressure as they try to care for the large volume of patients affected by COVID-19. In the ICUs, care provided is highly technical, fast paced, and involves intense 1-to-1 care where life and death is uncertain. In addition to the work related stresses and pressures FHP experience in regard to their jobs, they are also dealing with the fear of contracting the virus themselves and/or passing it on to their significant others. This day-in and day-out stress and pressure took its toll on these FHP. However, outward signs of the effects of this prolonged stress is not always visible and may not manifest itself until after a pandemic subsides. Much like a soldier returning and experiencing posttraumatic stress. The potential is there for these FHP to experience the same symptoms in the future.

Therefore, it is the responsibility of those healthcare facilities/institutions to provide avenues for these professionals to be able to connect and release these emotions. The environment resulting from attempts to contain and control viral spread, while providing care to those who are sick, created challenges these FHP have not previously experienced. At least not at this level of intensity and volume. This further reinforces the need for other strategies to be developed to assist FHP to cope with the situations they are facing on a daily basis during a pandemic.

Fear, stress and the many unknowns associated with this virus weighed heavy on the physical and mental health of FHP. The receipt of inconsistent and/or contradictory messaging from state and federal governments, as well as from their own healthcare facilities/institutions further complicated the situation. Messaging in the beginning of the pandemic focused on the availability of PPE rather on the development of best practices for dealing with the virus. This resulted in a drastic change in the normal process of care in the ICUs further contributing to the level of stress and anxiety experienced by FHP. These professionals struggled with interpersonal conflict in regard to their duty to provide care and the fear for their own safety as well as their safety of their significant others. However, one way to mitigate this interpersonal conflict is through coaching as a compliment to other strategies if employed by healthcare facilities/institutions. The use of coaching is one example of considering alternatives to connect with those at the frontlines of the pandemic response.

Those healthcare professionals at the front lines of the COVID-19 pandemic needed ongoing support to prevent uninterrupted patient care and staff burnout. The burnout experienced comes from a variety of avenues such as physical and emotional exhaustion and feelings of disconnection from the significance of what they are doing. Therefore, it is important to develop innovative strategies to help sustain FHP, helping them to assign personal, clinical and structural meaning to their work. In order to achieve this, it requires healthcare facilities/institutions to provide alternative resources/sources to help these essential individuals address their mental and physical health needs (Akgün et al., 2020).

FHP were not only a valuable resource during the COVID-19 pandemic; they remain a valuable resource for future health events as well. Therefore, it is important to learn from those first-hand experiences and make a commitment to "do better" in regard to taking care of those individuals at the frontlines of a pandemic. Engaging with those FHP is essential to help them deal with the immense stress, anxiety and fear they experienced. This includes coming up with alternative methods to connect with these individuals. Coaching is one of these methods, and when utilized on the front lines, affords FHP easier access to someone who will listen and assist them to process the events they are witnessing and are participating. Access to video coaching can also provide FHP help to work through the interpersonal conflicts they may be experiencing.

On the frontlines of pandemic patient care, a humanistic approach to coaching would help under these unique and intense circumstances. A humanistic coaching perspective aims to help expand individuals from merely functioning, to a level of understanding and emotional release, with the techniques and skills acquired applicable to an individual's personal and professional lives. While coaching focuses on actions as opposed to an individual's feelings, in a humanistic coaching approach, the goal is to increase an individual's clarity and awareness of a situation/experience and how that it is affecting them. This would afford frontline healthcare professionals an opportunity to find substance and meaning in the care they provide. Something they are struggling to connect with mentally and physically.

Another way to achieve this is to have a strategic staffing plan. Staff in areas that are operating at a reduced capacity may offer additional staff to reduce the burden in other areas. They can also offer expertise for highly complex cases making it easier to obtain consultations when needed. For those healthcare professionals reassigned from their typical units, the provision of training and resources prior to deployment will help alleviate the stress and anxiety of providing care on a floor or in an unfamiliar unit. For those older or at risk healthcare professionals, reassignment to supporting roles would provide support for those providing direct patient care by taking on such tasks as providing telephonic support for families of the patients receiving care while affording these workers a layer of protection. Ordering supplies and going to get meals are also support functions these personnel could do (Akgün, et al., 2020).

In addition, it becomes important for healthcare facilities/institutions in a particular area to collaborate in an effort to share information, resources and support one another. The use of technology and social networking resources can connect FHP with other facilities providing quicker access to needed expertise and information. Best practice information sharing along with clinical insights and similar experiences connect individuals in similar situations. This connection affords an opportunity to combat feelings of loneliness experienced by FHP (Akgün, et al., 2020).

The caring of patients with COVID-19 in and of itself was a challenge. The typical provision of bedside care was impeded by isolations rooms, multiple layers of PPE and the ever presence of loss of life. This continual negativism affected both the mental and physical health of FHP. These individuals needed, but often are not able to, take time to care for themselves. Facilities/institutions need to take a proactive approach to helping these FHP. They need time to reflect and talk about what they are seeing and feeling. They need to feel like their work is making a difference and to verbalize the challenges and pain they are experiencing. This can be accomplished by offering virtual support groups or virtual coaching. A chaplain or social worker trained in this area may be a good resource to host these sessions. Use of techniques such as mindfulness may also help FHP manage their stress and anxiety (Akgün, et al., 2020).

Other ideas to sustain FHP include virtual social gatherings so they can connect with individuals outside the hospital setting in the community. However, because of the emotional and physical toil long shifts can have on individuals, they often neglect themselves and do not reach out for help. Therefore, strategies to engage FHP should be easily accessible and not require much effort to engage in. Things such as free lunches, virtual dinners and/or happy hours might provide an easy and effective outlet. The offering of multiple avenues for connecting increase the likelihood FHP will engage (Akgün et al., 2020).

The need to develop strategies to alleviate the stress, fear and anxiety FHP are experiencing as they provide care for patients during a pandemic is essential to increase their ability to endure current events now and events in the future. The requirements facing these FHP as they care for the increasing number of patients, and the unfortunate percentage of deaths associated with the virus, takes a toll on the mental and physical health of these healthcare professionals. Without consideration of the need to address these concerns, the potential for long-term effects significantly increases. FHP experience emotional exhaustion and job burnout as they attempt to cope with the patient care aspects associated with caring for individuals with COVID-19. The unpreparedness and associated unknowns increases the likelihood a negative outcome will result in regard to the mental and physical health of these essential professionals as stress and exhaustion build to critical levels.

FHP are an essential resource to the provision of patient care and to the success of reigning in the current pandemic. Therefore, it is important to consider the needs of FHP in real time, as well as to consider the needs of these same individuals post-COVID. FHP will be needed postpandemic to provide patient care to those who are sick or injured. Taking steps now to help alleviate the emotional and physical effects COVID patient care is having on FHP during the pandemic will insure they will be able to care for patients postpandemic.

Without attention to these essential professionals during a pandemic, healthcare resources postpandemic has the potential for a reduction as the emotional and physical toll causes healthcare professionals to leave the industry/profession. Therefore, it is important to develop avenues to sustain these professionals not only through a pandemic and into the postpandemic period as well. The future effects of the COVID-19 pandemic on FHP is yet to be determined and remains essentially unknown. However, by taking proactive steps, healthcare facilities/institutions can help to insure a viable work force for patient care is available both during and postpandemic periods. FHP are a vital and scarce resource needed in the provision of patient care. Without efforts initiated to help them, and to incorporate the lessons learned from the COVID-19 pandemic, there is the potential for a reduced availability of these resources for the future.

REFERENCES

Akgün, K. M., Collett, D., Feder, S. L., Shamas, T., & Schulman-Green, D. (2020). Sustaining frontline ICU healthcare workers during the COVID-19 pandemic and beyond. *Heart & Lung, 49(2020)*, 346–347. https://www.ncbi.nlm.nih.gov/pmc/articles/PMC7256543/

Dawson, A., Isaacs, D., Jansen, M., Jordens, C., Kerridge, I., Kihlbom, U., Kilham, H., Preisz, A., Sheahan, L., & Skowronski, G. (2020). An ethics framework for making resource allocation decisions within clinical care: Responding to COVID-19. *Journal of Bioethical Inquiry, 17*, 1–7. https://link.springer.com/article/10.1007/s11673-020-10007-w

Dirani, K. M., Abadi, M., Alizadeh, A., Barhate, B., Garza, R. C., Gunasekara, N., Ibrahim, G., & Majzun, Z. (2020). Leadership competencies and the essential role of human resource development in times of crisis: A response to COVID-19 pandemic. *Human Resource Development International, 23(4)*, 329–467. https://www.tandfonline.com/doi/full/10.1080/13678868.2020.1780078

Emanuel, E., Persad, G., Upshur, R., Thome, B., Parker, M., Glickman, A., Zhang, C., Boyle, C., Smith, M., & Phillips, J. P. (2020). Fair allocation of scarce medical resources in the time of COVID-19. *New England Journal of Medicine, 382*(21), 2049–2055. https://www.nejm.org/doi/full/10.1056/NEJMsb2005114

Gereffi, G. (2020). What does the COVID-19 pandemic teach us about global value chains? The case of medical supplies. *Journal of International Business Policy, 3,* 287–301. https://link.springer.com/article/10.1057/s42214-020-00062-w

Guttman, N., & Lev, E. (2021). Ethical issues in COVID-19 communication to mitigate the pandemic: Dilemmas and practical implications. *Health Communication, 36*(1), 116–123. https://www.tandfonline.com/doi/full/10.1080/10410236.2020.1847439

Li, J. Y., Sun, R., Tao, W., & Lee, Y. (2021). Employee coping with organizational change in the face of a pandemic: The role of transparent internal communication. *Public Relations Review, 47,* 1–11.

McCullough, L. B. (2020). In response to COVID-19 pandemic physicians already know what to do. *The American Journal of Bioethics, 20*(7), 9–12. https://www.tandfonline.com/doi/pdf/10.1080/15265161.2020.1754100

Nicola, M., Alsafi, Z., Sohrabi, C., Kerwan, A., Al-Jabir, A., Iosifidis, C., Agha, M., & Agha, R. (2020). The socio-economic implications of the coronavirus pandemic (COVID-19): A review. *International Journal of Surgery, 78,* 185–193. https://www.ncbi.nlm.nih.gov/pmc/articles/PMC7162753/

Rawlings, A., Brandt, L., Ferreres, A., Asbun, H., & Shadduck, P. (2020). Ethical considerations for allocation of scarce resources and alterations in surgical care during a pandemic. *Surgical Endoscopy, 35,* 1–6. https://www.ncbi.nlm.nih.gov/pmc/articles/PMC7216853/

Schoch-Spana, M., Brunson, E. K., Gwon, H., Regenberg, A., Toner, E. S., & Daugherty-Biddison, E. L. (2020). Influence of community and culture in the ethical allocation of scarce medical resources in a pandemic situation: Deliberative democracy study. *Journal of Participatory Medicine, 12*(1), 1–14. https://jopm.jmir.org/2020/1/e18272

CHAPTER 4

THE PANDEMIC AND THE LONG-TERM UNEMPLOYED

A Road Map for a Job Search Turnaround

S. Charles Malka and Robert H. Tiell

COVID-19 has made an already precarious situation much worse for many employment seekers. The massive disruptions caused by the pandemic has slowed down the economy and triggered the shutdowns of businesses large and small. The tide of layoffs hit millions and has yet to subside. One particular group that has been hit the hardest consists of the long-term unemployed. Competing for work against those who recently lost their jobs may lead many long-term unemployed (LTU) to view their chances for landing satisfactory employment as further reduced, while others may have given up and are no longer seeking work. A common measure used by the U.S. Bureau of Labor Statistics (BLS) defines a LTU person as an individual who experienced a job separation lasting 27 weeks or more. Thus, by definition, you are considered LTU if you were separated from the labor force for at least 6 months.

Just how widespread is this dire problem? BLS estimates that at the end of 2020, close to 40% of unemployed people, or over 4 million, were out of work for 6 months or longer (BLS, 2021). *The Wall Street Journal*

Back to a New Normal: In Search of Stability in an Era of Pandemic Disruption—Insight From Practitioners and Academics, pp. 45–59

reported that the current size of people in this category represents the largest share of the unemployed since 2013 ("U.S. Employers Added," 2021). Undoubtedly, this is an unwelcomed blow exacerbated by the pandemic that bears heavily on the well-being of millions of individuals and their families. And, while economists expect job growth to pick up with a rise in vaccinations and business reopening, many of the unemployed may be discouraged by limited job opportunities, while others are occupied with child-care responsibilities, and still others are simply fearful of contracting the virus and opting to stay put for now. Against this background, we take a new second look at the unemployment phenomenon, with a focus on the LTU.

Consider that while the study of human work and the workplace occupies a central place in scientific thought and discourse, relatively less attention has been given to the unemployment phenomenon and far less to the long-term unemployment experience (Malka & Tiell, 2016). Therefore, we devote this chapter to members of this neglected large group, as well as to career service providers and other practitioners in the field. We offer some scientific-based observations as to the nature of unemployment and its health related implications, and highlight a possible interplay among unemployment relevant processes that bear on the individual's job search activities. We view these processes as interconnected components, or anchors, that shape the individual's state of mind and job search activity during the unemployment experience. For the practitioner in the employment field, the anchors—personal resources, infliction points, attitudes, incentives, and community-based programs—represent a five-legged stool upon which rests a viable assessment of needs and an effective intervention that is tailored to the LTU.

You may envision these anchors as being key markers on a road; using them as a diagnostic tool, facilitates assessment and allow for a personalized intervention. We consider our five-legged stool and the diagnostic model as additional items in the toolbox of employment counselors. In short, whether you are LTU, or a practitioner in a relevant field, we hope you find the information contained of interest to you.

THE SCENE: SHOW ME THE NUMBERS

To put things in perspective, let us compare current unemployment numbers with numbers from a few years ago, say 2015. The U.S Department of Labor estimated the jobless rate to stand at 5.0% in December of 2015. In December 2020, the unemployment rate stood at 6.7%. When we focus on the LTU, the comparative numbers are as significant; about one third of this group, or 1.8 million Americans, have been out of work for a year

Figure 4.1

Labor Force Participation in the United States

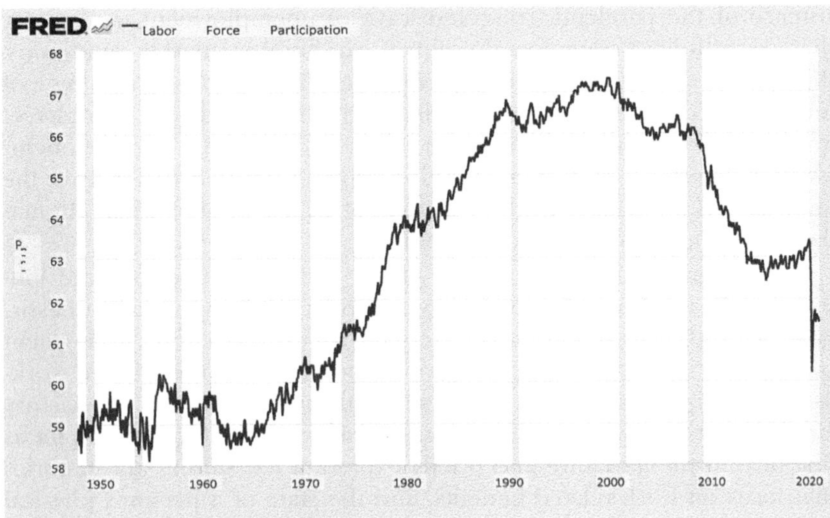

Source: U.S. Bureau of Labor (2021).

or more in 2015 (BLS, 2015). In January 2021, that number approached 4 million. No doubt, the pandemic had and continues to have a devastating effects on large swaths of employment seekers, and particularly on the LTU. The employment picture is still unclear if one tries to peer into the near future. Looking at it from a different angle, the numbers suggest that the total workforce participation rate that has been gradually declining in recent years, has dramatically accelerated since the pandemic hit. Figure 4.1 offers interesting insights.

Consider the continuous decline in total workforce participation taking place since the late 1990s, and note the remarkable drop that has taken place during 2020. Here too, a 3.1 percentage point drop from about 63.3 down to 60.2 during a single year can be clearly attributed to one dramatic event that occurred in 2020—the pandemic. And since the labor force participation rate reflects the sum of employed and unemployed persons, you can easily conclude that while the LTU are accounted for, the radical drop in labor force participation also reflects the simple fact that many have given up for various reasons and are no longer seeking employment. Given that labor force participation is a driver of economic growth, encouraging and assisting the unemployed, and particularly the

LTU, with their job search activities serves both individual needs and larger community goals, as well as the economy as a whole.

Optimists among us may argue that despite the magnitude and persistence of the pandemic-triggered wave of unemployment, a recovery that always follows economic downturns can improve market conditions, thus reducing the ranks of the unemployed. If one follows the logic of improved economy and increased labor demand, would it be also correct to assume that employers may turn first to workers with shorter unemployment spells? If such an assumption proves correct, it would leave the unemployed pool increasingly composed of LTU who are socially stigmatized and whose work skills keep eroding.

Several questions may come to mind. Just how important are job-search skills for those who still seek work? Specifically, what kind of assistance and guidance should career service professionals and employment counselors extend the LTU? And, what role can community-based workforce organizations play for those who still hope to land a satisfactory employment? We address these questions later in this chapter. But, let us first turn to the literature and briefly explore a few studies and theories that focus on work related benefits, and the state of a person's physical and cognitive health during an extended period of separation from work.

RESEARCH BITES: WHAT DO WE KNOW?

Generally speaking, we know that unemployment carries profound effects and implications for individuals and their communities, and bears negatively on the economy as a whole. Research stresses the negative impact of job loss on individuals' health, financial distress, obsolescence of skills, depleted social network, mortality rate, precautionary savings, and welfare. Such negative effects are well documented (Carlier et al., 2013; Krug & Eberl, 2018). Similarly, research has employed a host of general psychology and career theories in an effort to study numerous unemployment related constructs. A partial list includes a sense of coherence following job loss (Vastamaki, 2009), job-search persistence (Wanberg et al., 2005), self-efficacy (Albion et al., 2005), locus of control (Creed et al., 2012; van Hooft & Crossley, 2008), and self-determination and job flexibility (Broeck et al., 2010).

As you can tell, a long list of job loss related aspects has been scientifically explored. But, surprisingly, only partial attention was given by this stream of studies to the LTU, and to contingency (i.e., situational) variables capable of influencing the job loss-job search and reemployment relationship. Is there an explanation for the insufficient interest shown in the literature toward a growing subgroup of the unemployed population?

Are there relevant theories dedicated to the LTU? Is there a place for a theory that offers insight into the process of job-search by LTU?

It is somewhat disappointing to find out that little is reported with regard to our target group. For instance, notable theories that were developed for the specific study of the effects of unemployment on an individual's well-being, such as Jahoda's latent deprivation theory (1981), Fryer's agency theory (1995), and Warr's vitamin model (1987), do not directly address the LTU. All three theories provide sound insights into psychological processes that highlight the individual's state of well-being following job loss, but none addresses the processes relative to the experience of job search among the LTU as a group.

Let's zoom in on these theories just a bit more:

- Jahoda's latent deprivation theory (1981) was developed within the context of unemployment and suggested that job loss deprived the unemployed of manifest and latent benefits. Jahoda explained that aside from the loss of income, individuals are deprived of time structure, social contact, activity, identity and shared purpose. Such benefit deprivation negatively affects a person's mental health and well-being.
- In contrast to Jahoda's deprivation theory, Fryer (1995) advanced an agency theory and argued that the five stated latent benefits of employment are claimed to often be costs of employment rather than benefits. In other words, a bad job carries the risk of affecting individuals' mental health more than no job or unemployment per se.
- Warr's (1987) Vitamin model is concerned with the effects of certain environmental features on mental health. Warr suggested that nine features of the environment have a curvilinear effect on mental health, similar to the way vitamins influence physical health. Among the features that work provides are the opportunity for control, skill use, generated goals, money, physical security, and social position. Without suggesting that employment is necessarily better than unemployment in terms of these nine features, the model leads one to assume that unlike the state of unemployment, the work experience tends to provide these features at beneficial levels.

You may be correct to conclude that an assessment of the three theories yields little insight, if any, into the LTU experience and into the dynamics of the job-search process per se. And, you may be wondering as to the reason for the limited attention given this particular group. We propose that the apparent partial empirical curiosity with long-term unemployment, and the little interest manifested by the paucity of community-based initiatives and intervention programs (that we note later), may well be attributed to a dominant ideological view that perceives long-term unemployment to be an individual matter rather than a larger social issue. It is even more likely that researchers and practitioners alike don't see a significant difference between short- and long-term unemployment and thus see no need for separate programs and investigations targeting these respective populations.

Moving away from the realm of theory and empiricism into the domain of government, shifts the attention to managed and funded programs for the unemployed. Reviewing the gamut of government programs that are relevant to the unemployed is beyond the scope of this chapter. Instead, we are curious about the overall effectiveness of these programs; Are they being administered properly? Is their coordination done efficiently? How about impact studies concerning program outcomes? Any notable duplication and waste?

A GOVERNMENT HELPING HAND: IS THERE MUCH TO SHARE?

Here are a few observations. A government helping hand thus far has done little to alleviate the plight of the unemployed brought about by the pandemic. 2020 saw a government sponsored program for businesses in the form of a paycheck protection program (PPP). This program was designed to provide a temporary relief allowing businesses to hold on to their employees to minimize layoffs. Thus, the PPP program skipped those who have been unemployed before the pandemic hit. And aside from the PPP, the government introduced several rounds of direct payments for all that gradually phased out at various income levels. The limited payments were likely to have a small effect on the unemployed. Only scant data is available about other programs that put people, and especially the LTU back to work. Consider an earlier General Accountability Office (GAO) report made public in 2011; it suggested that of the 49 federal job training programs administered by nine agencies and costing about $14.5 billion in 2010, only five have had impact studies aimed at establishing rates of improvement in employment outcomes. The audit further determined that the effect the five programs had on employment outcomes was only negligibly positive, inconclusive, or restricted to short term impact (GAO, 2011). The effectiveness and efficiency in delivery of services by the other 44 federal programs remained unknown.

A decade later, a GAO report made public in 2019 reported similar findings. Little has changed. In fact, there was a reduction in the number of programs for the unemployed, down to 43 from 47, and a reduction in funding. The report points to the lack of coordination among available employment and training programs, with multiple programs providing similar services to similar groups of people. And, still a scant number of impact studies were carried out, similar to the few reported a decade earlier. Waste and inefficiencies remain rampant (GAO, 2019).

As surprising is the paucity of intervention programs designed for the LTU at state and community levels. A decade ago, Katz (2010) mentioned in testimony to Congress only a few community-based sectoral employment programs that help connect job seekers with local and regional employers. However, little has changed since then. Consider that a recent survey of directors of career service providers across the U.S., conducted in late 2016, found no documented programs that specifically targeted the LTU population (Malka & Tiell, 2016).

And so, what can be done? We argue that interventions designed to assist the LTU in securing a job before structural barriers take root are warranted. They ought to be considered by public policy makers and by workforce development administrators at the state level. We also argue that effective vehicles for change include community-based career service providers. And, we believe that while any sponsored program or empirical inquiry on unemployment can be applied to short-term as well as long-term unemployment, members of the latter group deserve special attention given their greater vulnerability in terms of resource deficit and well-being.

The U.S. Congress Joint Economic Committee's report on long-term unemployment, concluded some years ago that as job searches drag on, skills atrophy and social networks fade, thus making it more difficult for this particular population to find work. The report further argues that given the rapid pace of technological advancements and shifts in high-growth sectors of the economy, the location of, and the knowledge and skills required for tomorrow's jobs are less likely to be found among the LTU (U.S. Congress Joint Economic Committee, 2013). As suggested earlier, we devote the balance of the discussion to a framework that rests on five components, or anchors, around which career service practitioners can tailor responsive intervention plans geared to meet the needs of the LTU.

THE FRAMEWORK: HOW RELEVANT ARE THE ANCHORS?

Our framework rests on five anchors capable of influencing the long-term unemployment-job search-reemployment relationship: *Resource scarcity, time as an infliction point, job-search attitudes, government incentives, and community-based job search programs*. We briefly discuss each component and highlight their relevance to the LTU sustainability and job search activity. We contend that our framework when applied to a proposed matrix model, presented next, can form the basis for an effective intervention by career service providers on behalf of the LTU.

Resource Scarcity. The level of a person's resources is highly relevant as it determines the individual's ability to endure downturns such as a layoff, and shapes job search activity. The personal resources of the LTU, their human capital, social capital and psychological capital are perceived as ability enhancers when coping with life stressors such as a job loss.

Also consider that personal resources can play an important role in reducing the adverse effects of job-search setbacks, as well as in broadening access to employment opportunities, and thus as possible factor of one's employability (De Cuyper, 2012). Human capital refers to education and learned skills and past and present work experience; social capital refers to social relationships that can confer influence and provide access to external resources and information; and psychological capital refers to one's sense of mastery and control critical and conducive to decision making.

If we entertain a relevant theory that sheds light on subject matter, Hobfoll's theory of conservation of resources (Hobfoll, 1989) appears particularly relevant for understanding the potential role resources can play during unemployment. Hobfoll defines resources as valued factors that meet survival needs of the individual. This theory posits that individuals flourish when they gain, maintain and conserve resources. The addition of resources means enhanced survival capabilities. More resources allow the individual to compartmentalize stress following loss and setbacks, augment resiliency, and accommodate, withstand and overcome threats. On the other hand, stressful or traumatic events consume such resources and increase sensitivity to subsequent stressors. Applied to the LTU, job loss triggers heightened stressors that negatively affect resources, as well as, some personal characteristics with the passing of time, such as work skills.

Infliction Point. Time as a critical factor is relevant as well. The probable impact of time on the human, social, and psychological capital of the LTU cannot be ignored, and should be carefully considered when evaluating individual resource inventory and sustainability, and when considering assessment and intervention. We apply the concept of infliction point to highlight the critical importance of time and use the term somewhat loosely to illustrate a possible association between time and personal resources.

Given the finite nature of resources, the longer a person is unemployed the greater the probability of personal resources being consumed with the passing of time. Some degree of resource loss, beyond the sheer loss of income, characterizes a person's experiences during varying periods of unemployment.

Understand that as individual resources are invested and consumed in job search, they reach a point beyond which further drops in human, social, and psychological capital may undermine the individual's welfare and well-being. The unemployed's coping resources can also reach the infliction point. Ideally, reemployment and/or professional intervention should occur prior to a person reaching their infliction point. Practitioners, therefore, needs to aim at reinforcing the individual's personal resource inventory, thereby assisting in changing the possible trajectory of decline and reversing its direction toward personal sustainability, adaptation and growth.

A practitioner may well be aware of changes in the dynamics of search behaviors that occur with the passing of time. A bit dated but still a relevant work, Sharone (2007) found periods of boost and bust that characterize job seekers with the passing of time. Namely, an initial phase of energetic engagement and a burst of activity devoted to the task of job searching, and a second phase characterized by self-blame as confidence in job search strategy erodes with reoccurring employer rejection over time.

We contend that given the probable shifts in emotions and cognitions, and the individual's reactions to unemployment with the passing of time, pursuing intervention options that range from fine-tuning job search practices to renewing self-confidence and augmenting resources appears critical for the unemployed, and are particularly warranted in the case of the LTU.

Attitudes. A person's overall attitude toward their unemployment experience and job search is perhaps one of the most relevant factors to be considered. The impact of attitudes on job search intentions and behavior occupies a central place in several works (e.g., Lopez-Kidwell et al., 2013; Wanberg, et al., 2010). At the heart of this stream of research lies the theory of planned behavior (TPB). This theory asserts that behavior is explained by a person's intention (Ajzen, 1991). Antecedents of the latter are the person's attitudes toward the behavior (e.g., favorable or unfavorable appraisal of the behavior), the subjective norm (e.g., social pressure from significant others relative to the behavior), and the perceived behavioral control (e.g., perceived difficulty in performing the behavior).

Just how relevant is the theory of planned behavior to the LTU? The theory of planned behavior suggests that a positive assessment of self-performance of a particular behavior (e.g., job-search) refers to a belief that job search, as a proposed *"preventive behavior,"* reduces the vulnerability to the negative outcomes of unemployment. This in turn leads others (e.g., family members, friends) to view such behavior positively, and the individual's perceived control over it increases given cognitive traits such as locus of control and other well studied dispositions of job seekers.

Consider that an internal self-control reflects the individual's perception of unemployment as being controllable by one's capacity to engage in active search routines, thus viewing one's state of unemployment as a temporary rather than a permanent phase, and thereby positively affecting the individual's search routine. Such realization opens up opportunities for professional intervention aimed at reinforcing the perception of controllability by the individual.

External government incentives. Interestingly, some government incentives have turned into a thorny issue in public discourse at the midst of the current pandemic (e.g., Rampell, 2020). How damaging are increased unemployment insurance payments? Unemployment insurance and other incentives in the form of governmental benefit payments are critical in the aftermath of a job loss. Yet, such incentives are reported to be positively linked to the duration of unemployment.

External incentives coupled with a weak labor demand were found to be the prime drivers of the dramatic rise in the average duration of unemployment (Aaronson et al, 2010). Aaronson et al., suggested that government extensions in unemployment benefits emerged as a significant factor that exacerbated such rise. The negative impact of external incentives on job search was likewise reported by studies outside the United States (McDonald & Marston, 2008). Overall, research suggests that unemployment benefit receipt undermine labor market participation and job search activities (Lazear, 2013). Limited in time, such incentives may not be available to long-term job seekers.

Community-based job search programs. Research suggests that counseling and job search assistance are the most effective forms of intervention with the unemployed (Thomsen, 2009). Research evidence also suggests that community-based programs prove to be more effective and less expensive in providing such interventions compared with other traditional training programs. Given their advantage in terms of proximity, agile structure and responsiveness, community-based organizations appear to be better positioned to counsel the unemployed.

Calls for the creation of a structural market for community-based providers of counseling and advice that target the unemployed go back as far as a decade ago (Katz, 2010). Those providers are envisioned to supplement poorly accessible and fragmented governmental services, thus the importance of community-based interventions, in terms of access and content, cannot be understated.

PUTTING IT ALL TOGETHER: ARE THE ANCHORS REAL ROAD MARKERS?

The combined effect of the five anchors is critical as it shapes the overall experience of the unemployed and governs the ability, intensity, and duration of their job search activity. Equally important is the ability of a helping practitioner to adequately assess the weight of each anchor, and the way they may be leveraged. For the LTU, an expedient community-based professional response is critical in light of crucial infliction points, a change in attitudes, and depletion of personal resources regardless of government incentives. Thus, the identified anchors serve as a road map for practitioners by establishing a baseline from which a professional intervention can start.

Interventions that benefit the LTU may be guided by one or more of the following empirically grounded themes:

A targeted investment in *personal control and efficacy* through cognitive reframing and behavior modification, thereby strengthening resiliency of individuals with low self-efficacy and locus of control, and thereby increasing effective job search behavior.

- A targeted investment in the *reorientation of the individual's work value* system, by reducing job-seekers extrinsic work value orientation in favor of an intrinsic one, thereby increasing individual's job-flexibility.
- A targeted investment in the *unemployed who express employment intentions*, thereby supporting active job search behavior.
- And, a targeted investment in *competence and social network* thereby positively affecting job-seeking behavior and increased employment probability.

Guided by the empirically grounded themes, Figure 2 depicts a multi-level intervention model that can guide employment counseling and job-placement practitioners when dealing with the LTU. Building on Noer's (1993) work, we applied a multilevel intervention typology to a matrix model that incorporates both an intervention depth with the breadth of issues to be dealt with.

This model highlights the importance of identifying and dealing with the host of resource deficits, infliction points, and behaviors that are expressed, suppressed, and acted out following job loss. Let's touch briefly on each block in the model:

- *Grieving intervention* focuses narrowly but with great depth on the most pressing active-destructive behaviors, such as anger and aggression that the LTU may exhibit. This intervention seeks to ensure that latent and salient destructive behaviors do not intensify with time.

- *Process intervention* targets secondary symptoms and behaviors that are passive-destructive, such as apathy and depression. Process intervention, using less breadth and depth, seeks to minimize risks, and its ultimate goal is to help move the LTU toward a fuller functioning.
- *Empowerment intervention* leverages the unemployed repertoire of resources, considering resource deficits and inflection points, aimed at regaining a sense of control. With great depth and intensity, this intervention helps the unemployed rebuild diminished resources, explore setback inoculation options, and prepare for a job search turnaround.
- Finally, *Systems intervention*, educational and informational driven, seeks to disseminate vital information about other support systems that can further assist the LTU. This intervention level, broad in scope but limited in depth and intensity, informs individuals of other existing government incentives and community-based resources.

You may find the intervention themes and the practical model of value. As you reflect on the model's merit and possible use, also consider some cautionary advice. Notwithstanding the model's integrative qualities, Figure 4.2 presents some challenges for practitioners.

- First, managing a multilevel intervention process, at times simultaneously, is a complex task to consider.
- Second, determining the breadth of issues to be captured and the depth with which they ought to be approached is another critical task to be contemplated.

Figure 4.2

Multilevel Intervention Model

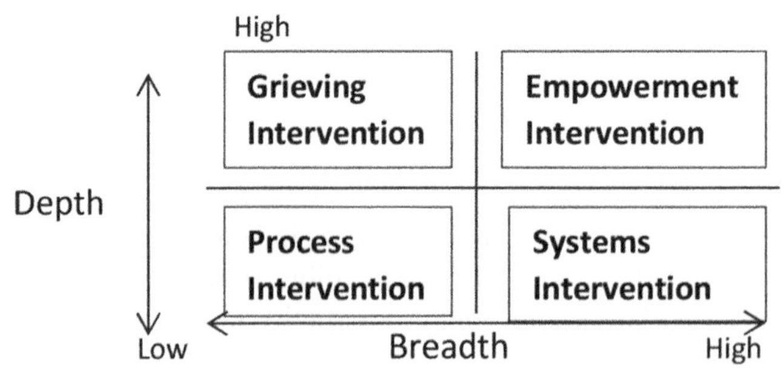

- Third, in light of agency resource constraints, prioritizing targets for intervention requires careful evaluation and assessment of at-risk groups. A targeted investment in a LTU group with strong job search intentions may be one initial option to explore.
- Fourth, the level of program customization within areas of individual resource scarcity and infliction points should also dictate who should be targeted first by an intervention. Ultimately, the choice is primarily between those LTU who are most vulnerable in terms of coping resource deficit, and those who are actively engaged in job search activities, thus being more motivated to reenter the labor force. An effective action is for a practitioner to first target subgroups that carry higher promise such as the active job seeker and those with strong employment intentions.
- Finally, adding practical potency to some of the proposed conceptual mapping tools in our article requires the development of related metrics. Absent such quantifying measures, infliction points, job search attitudes, resource inventory audits and intervention themes while conceptually meaningful will remain wanting in terms of practical applicability.

EPILOGUE: THE LAST WORD?

The current pandemic has thrown millions into a state of unemployment, a dysfunctional event that affects the mental and physical health of individuals and families. Of those, more than 40% are defined as LTU by the U.S. Bureau of Labor Statistics (2021). COVID-19 exacerbated the misfortunes of many that may have been unemployed before the pandemic hit. The ferocity of the virus and the disruptions it caused the economy are likely to continue well into the near future and trigger business cycle fluctuations, occupational and technology changes in the form of AI and automation.

Such changes are likely to worsen the unemployment numbers, and exacerbate the rate of decline in labor force participation thus curtailing a driving force of economic growth. For practitioners in the field, the growth in the ranks of this population presents a challenge. Left unattended, a polarized labor market may emerge with a growing class of alienated and displaced workers whose skills erode with the passing of time.

At the same time, the pandemic opens up an opportunity for change. It may well accelerate a paradigm shift in the employment environment that has been under way. Such a shift mandates the abandonment of the job-for-life contract for a short-term contingency driven one, further fueling the gig economy. And may propel further the transfer of responsibility for job stability, career development and growth to the individual.

AUTHORS' NOTE

This is a modified version of S. C. Malka and R. Tiell (2016), "Job search turnaround and the long-term unemployed: An exploratory framework and a contingency model," *Vocational Evaluation and Career Assessment Professionals Journal, 11*(1), 9–26. Used and modified with permission.

REFERENCES

Aaronson, D., Mazumder, B., & Schechter, S. (2010). What is behind the rise in long term unemployment? *Economic perspectives*. Federal Reserve Bank.

Ajzen, I. (1991). The theory of planned behavior. *Organizational Behavior and Human Decision Processes, 50,* 179–211.

Albion, J. M., Fernie, M. K., & Burton, J. L. (2005). Individual differences in age and self-efficacy in the unemployed. *Australian Journal of Psychology, 57*(1), 11–19.

Broeck, A. V., Vansteenkiste, M., Lens, W., & De Witte, H. (2010). Unemployed individuals' work values and job flexibility: An explanation from expectancy-value theory and self-determination theory. *Applied Psychology: An International Review*. *59*(2), 296–317.

Carlier, E. B., Schuring, M., Lotters, J. F., Bakker, B., Borgers, N., & Burdorf, A. (2013). The influence of re-employment on quality of life and self-rated health, a longitudinal study among unemployed persons in the Netherlands. *BMC Public Health, 13*, 503, 1–7.

Creed, P. A., Hood, M., & Leung, L. Y. (2012). The relationship between control, job Seeking, and well-being in unemployed people. *Journal of Applied Social psychology, 42*(3), 689–701.

De Cuyper, N., Makikangas, A., Kinnunen, U., Mauno, S., & De Witte, H. (2012). Cross-lagged associations between perceived external employability, job insecurity, and exhaustion: Testing gain and loss spirals according to the conservation of resources theory. *Journal of Organizational Behavior, 33*, 770–788.

Fryer, D. M. (1995, June). Benefit agency? Labour market disadvantage, deprivation and mental health. *The Psycho*, 265–272.

General Accountability Office. (2011, January 21). *Multiple employment and training programs*, Report to Congressional Requesters.

General Accountability Office. (2019, March). *Employment and training programs: Department of Labor should assess efforts to coordinate services across programs* (GAO-19-200).

Hobfoll, S. E. (1989). Conservation of resources: A new attempt at conceptualizing stress. *American Psychologist. 44*, 513–524.

Jahoda, M. (1981). Work, employment and unemployment: Values, theories, and approaches in social research. *American Psychologist. 36*, 184–191.

Katz, F. L. (2010, April 29). *Long term unemployment in the Great Recession*. Testimony for the Joint Economic Committee. U.S. Congress.

Krug, G., & Eberl, A. (2018). What explains the negative effect of unemployment on health? An analysis accounting for reverse causality. *Research in Social Stratification and Mobility, 55,* 25–39.

Lazear, P. E. (2013, June 6). The hidden jobless disaster. *The Wall Street Journal,* Opinion page.

Lopez-Kidwell, V., Grosser, J. T., Dineen, R. B., and Borgatti, P. S. (2013). What matters when: A multistage model and empirical examination of job search effort. *Academy of Management Journal, 56*(6), 1655–1678.

Malka, S. M., & Tiell, R. (2016). Job search turnaround and the long term unemployed: An exploratory framework and a contingency model. *Vocational Evaluation and Career Assessment Professionals Journal, 11*(1), 9–26.

McDonald, C., & Marston, G. (2008). Motivating the unemployed? Attitudes at the front line. *Australian Social Work, 61*(4), 315–326.

Noer, M. D. (1993). *Healing the wounds: Overcoming the trauma of layoffs and revitalizing downsized.* Jossey-Bass.

Rampell, C. (2020; August 3). The myth of unemployment benefits depressing work. *The Washington Post,* p. D4.

Sharone, O. (2007). Constructing unemployed job seekers as professional workers: the depoliticizing work-game of job searching. *Qualitative Sociology, 30,* 403–416.

Thomsen, L. S. (2009). Explaining the employability gap of short term and long-term unemployed persons. *Kyklos, 2*(3), 448–478.

U.S. Bureau of Labor Statistics. (2015, April 3). The employment situation. News Release—USDL 15-0530.

U.S. Bureau of Labor Statistics. (2021, February 5). Unemployed persons by duration of unemployment. *Economic News Release,* Table A-12. https://www.bls.gov/news.release/empsit.t12.htm

U.S Congress, Joint Economic Committee. (2013, April). Long term unemployment in the U.S.

U.S. employers added 49,000 jobs in January. (2021, February 5). *The Wall Street Journal,* pp. A1–A2.

van Hooft, A. J. Edwin, & Crossley, D. C. (2008). The joint role of locus of control and perceived financial need in job search. *International Journal of Selection and Assessment, 16*(3), 258–271.

Vastamaki, J., Moser, K., & Paul, K. I. (2009). How stable is sense of coherence? Changes following an intervention for unemployed individuals. *Scandinavian Journal of Psychology, 50,* 161–171.

Wanberg, C. R., Glomb, T. M., Song, Z., & Sorenson, S. (2005). Job search persistence during unemployment: A 10-wave longitudinal study. *Journal of Applied Psychology, 90,* 411–430.

Wanberg, C., Zhu, J., & van Hooft, E. (2010). The job search grind: Perceived progress, self-reactions, and self-regulation of search effort. *Academy of Management Journal, 53,* 788–807.

Warr, P. B. (1987). *Work, unemployment, and mental health.* Clarendon.

CHAPTER 5

MONETIZING COMPASSION

The Case for a New-Age Currency

R. Brayton Bowen

PROLOGUE

Compassion is frequently associated with words like "mercy," "empathy," "caring," and "love." Words which in today's society seem to be of dubious value to some. By extension, our culture in the United States appears to be taking on the form of a "cultist" society, where the dismemberment of our culture into subgroups such as racial and religious minorities, political factions, sexual orientation, et cetera enables the leaders of the cult to maintain control. "Remote," "robotic," and "unemotional" are descriptors of the new workplace, as thousands of employees work remotely, and corporate landscapes reshape themselves to shed thousands more.

In the ravages of a global pandemic, the perils of "organizational distancing" are emerging and indeed intensifying, as the "distant" become more "inanimate" and less "precious." COVID-19 has forced people to seek shelter and to avoid assembling in public and traveling. The latter includes commuting via public transportation. Working from home has become the norm, and the closing of schools has made the distancing of workers from job sites even more pronounced, as workers tend to home

Back to a New Normal: In Search of Stability in an Era of Pandemic Disruption—Insight From Practitioners and Academics, pp. 61–84

schooling of their offspring. In the meantime, human resource parlance abounds with terms that sound more cerebral, more scientific, more intellectual. What is lost in all the blather is compassionate concern for those organizationally distanced and appreciation of the incredible value of their metaknowledge, compassionate leadership, and constructive organization cultures.

The French sociologist Émile Durkheim in his study on suicide discussed the concept of "anomie" or "anomy" as a condition of instability in societies or in individuals wherein there is a breakdown of standards and values or a lack of purpose or ideals. Any number of successful business organizations endeavor to create visions, mission statements and codes of conduct to keep employees engaged and companies profitable. They seek to embrace diversity, promote inclusion, and form cultures that are constructive, enterprising, collaborative, and self-actualizing. Unfortunately, the endeavors of these successful organizations are not particularly emulated by others. In my study of competencies of compassion, implementing seven specific competencies of compassion can positively impact the performance of an enterprise up to 40%, while engaging the passion of employees.

By contrast in a social system such as an organization that is in a state of anomie, common values and common meanings are no longer understood or accepted. Durkheim found in such societies many of its members developed psychological states characterized by a sense of futility, a lack of purpose, a loss of commitment, despondency, and despair. What is a common condition within many organizations is a concept that I choose to call "organizational distancing," where employees, working remotely and virtually, are "forgotten," in some fashion. Indeed, even those working within the organization are often treated like robots or dispensable commodities that can be furloughed, move about and terminated. Communication links between manager and the managed are weak, distant, unemotional, bland, perfunctory, et cetera. In such oases, where caring is a "mirage," any number of workers die of thirst, in a manner of speaking, for lack of appreciation and nurturance. Like strangers in the night the relationships are transient and are destined to wither and die.

Ironically, human resource professionals lament that employees are not "engaged" and that to retrain "good" employees, there needs to be effective "onboarding" and "engagement" efforts. This is true. But for the most part these professionals are more engaged in administrative tasks and compliance initiatives rather than the art of compassion. In the following chapter, I will explore the concept of competencies of compassion in the workplace, in fact, seven specific competencies that inspire employees, improve organizational performance, and increase profits up to 40%.

THE CASE FOR NEW-AGE CURRENCY

In the midst of what promises to be one of the worst pandemics in human history, most organizations are simply struggling to survive. Others are going under. First responders are risking their lives, while other wage earners—both salaried and hourly—from almost all segments of the economy are risking their health, their livelihood, and their careers. When the average American has to choose between putting food on the table and keeping the lights on; when living paycheck to paycheck is not helping ends meet; or, when people are subsisting on income that barely exceeds national poverty levels, the old way of "rewarding" people will not continue to work, if it ever did.

Moreover, the concept of work-life balance is changing, as workers reassess the benefits of working remotely versus working on-site. Working from home has its advantages, such as not having to dress for work; not having to pay launderers for cleaning business attire; not having to commute; not having to pay for daycare; not having to engage in office politics; et cetera. And even though any number of workers miss being able to socialize at work, the mood about working on-site versus working remotely is changing. Nearly 3 million U.S. women have dropped out of the workforce this past year, and any number are not wanting to return. The potential for the passage of certain administrative policies, such as subsidies for daycare could change that. But the odds are questionable. In the meantime, other factors are determinants in the assessment process, as we will discuss. They include the nature of the organization culture, the relationship with management, especially one's immediate supervisor, and the system of recognition and rewards.

On the other side of the employer/employee relationship is the matter of square footage. That's right, corporate overhead in the form of office space, property expense, maintenance, lease agreements, et cetera. Ford Motor Company just announced a new progressive, flexible, hybrid work model for its employees. The iconic automobile company plans to redesign the workplace radically. Some 30,000 white-collar office workers have been told they can continue to work from home "indefinitely" and they can have "flexible hours approved by their managers." It is anticipated that people will come into the office primarily for meetings and group projects.

Technology plays a key role in the decision to operate remotely. Zoom, Google Meet. and other software systems have stepped into the void of no face-to-face meetings. They are becoming familiar tools of communication in the office of the future. In the meantime, other organizations, including Google, Spotify, Salesforce, and Twitter, are making worker-friendly programs available. The workplace of the postpandemic era will look vastly different from that of the prepandemic age. Indeed, organizational distancing is on the rise and will be a phenomenon to deal with far into the future.

Suffice it to say, it is time to rethink the competencies of the organization. It's time to cut through the apathy of organizational distancing. It is time to revisit the traditional way of "doing business." It is time for a new "currency," one that fulfills the emotional, psychological, and economic needs of people; one that improves not only bottom-line performance and market reputation but also the quality of work life within organizational systems as a whole. I am referring to the "currency" of compassion. Is it possible to make money by implementing competencies of compassion in the workplace? Absolutely! Compassion can be monetized, as I will explain as we discuss the implementation of seven specific competences of compassion.

COMPASSION IN ACTION

In 1995 Aaron Feuerstein was the owner of Malden Mills, a factory in Lawrence, MA. The factory was destroyed by fire. More than 3,000 workers were without jobs. During the time the factory was being rebuilt, Feuerstein continued to pay them, with full benefits, for 6 months.

> I have a responsibility to the worker, both blue collar and white collar. I have an equal responsibility to the community. It would have been unconscionable to put 3,000 people on the streets and deliver a deathblow to the cities of Lawrence and Methuen. Maybe on paper our company is worthless to Wall Street, but I can tell you it's worth more. (Feuerstein, n.d.)

So, what did he buy, you might ask? Well, he bought the availability of an entire workforce and the loyalty of those he had led. Aaron Feuerstein was the quintessential steward, one would argue. He knew the value of the true assets of his company, namely the competencies and skills of his workers. Their return to work enabled Malden Mills to resume operations and land future contracts. Today the skills and competencies of those who have been furloughed and terminated have value, as they anxiously and prayerfully await return to work and/or look for new employment. Their familiarity with the businesses of their employers, known as "metaknowledge," makes ramping up even more expedient for those enterprises. And, as in legal settlements that include "pain and suffering," their time and talent should be valued. Moreover, as with distant relatives, it is important to stay in touch, even in the case of those who have been terminated. They are your "marketers" who can speak well of you if you treat them compassionately. Indeed, during dark times, compassion and caring are essential. An occasional call to ask: "How are you doing?" to say, "You are missed"; "We are looking forward to your return"; "Please stay well"; and "We wish every success." Even in these times of social distancing, exceptional efforts can and must be made to stay connected with one another. The story of Aaron Feuerstein is a story of leadership, stewardship, and human compassion.

The phrase "we are all in this together" has no meaning in the vacuum of deafening silence and inaction. A relative in an extended care facility welcomes hearing from family. A son who is undergoing treatment in another state wants to hear from a parent. The family that agonizes over being separate from a daughter who is giving birth to her first born makes every effort to make her aware of their love; prayers for her safety and well-being are sent her way. In the same manner, furloughed employees and others who are idled deserve to know they are valued. Those employees remaining in the trenches deserve to be recognized for their contributions. In the absence of compassion, one feels no connection, no commitment, no respect. And in return, business operators can be certain there is no personal commitment to stay on the job if unappreciated or once back on the job if invited to return. If a better opportunity comes along, the disenfranchised, the unrecognized, the unappreciated will be gone. Like strangers in the night, relationships are temporal. "There's no love lost," you might say, because there was no love. Independent parties that are not interdependent are not invested in the long haul. The enlightened leader regards herself or himself as caring, compassionate, and a "big-picture" thinker. Recognizing and rewarding employees compassionately pays off. So, a word to the wise. Care about your people. value their skills and competencies. Appreciate their uniqueness. Provide meaningful recognition and "new-age" rewards for those who toil in the trenches, and for those furloughed or terminated; should they return, value them as if they had never left.

In my research of organizations and institutions of all sorts—religious, political, professional, public and private, I have come to learn there are four relational dimensions that are held in common by followers, employees and customers alike: The first is *affinity*—the force that attracts people to enter into a relationship, or induces customers to buy services and products, or motivates employees to want to come to work. The second is *engagement*—the factor that prompts people to want to remain in association with organizations, or customers to continue to buy goods and services. The third factor is *disaffection*—the dissatisfaction that prompts people to want to leave relationships or to stop buying goods and services, perhaps because of the cost or quality, or because of insufficient appreciation, or poor leadership, or bad politics, or whatever else. And finally, there is the factor of *disinterest*—when people are apathetic about these relationships or when they do not want to be associated with an organization, for any number of reasons: poor management, questionable reputation, poor community relations, or just mundane performance. The challenge for thought-leaders, heads of business, and stewards of the economy is to innovate, differentiate, and invite all people, including customers, employees, and followers, into relationships that are mutually beneficial, regenerative, and even impassioned. We need to create systems that enlighten self-interest, where people are willing to risk the investment of themselves, along with their trust and personal dedication. And finally, as a society we need to eschew the conditions that cause people to lose faith in the very leaders and institutions that are responsible for their wellbeing, be it spiritual, physical, political, or financial.

This chapter provides basic information about the competencies of compassion, why compassion is so needed in our universe at this time, and what you need do to become a compassion advocate and a compassionate professional. To succeed it is necessary that you have a vision of what a "better world" would look like, whether at work or in the larger community. You will need to inspire others to join with you in fulfilling your vision. Next, you will need to understand the requirements for creating a constructive culture, one where others work together, collaborate, and cooperate to achieve fulfilling outcomes. Other areas of importance include: your values system; the ways in which members are recognized and rewarded; stewardship, the attribute of serving a larger universe; and engaging in socially responsible endeavors. So, let us begin with a brief discussion of why Compassion is important. Our assertion is that compassion is in fact the "new-age currency."

Organization Culture

There are various systems that enable one to determine organizational effectiveness. The metrics we use in our consultancy allows us to assess which elements are contributing to behaviors that encourage teamwork, improve decision-making, achieve better performance results, and respect the dignity of every organizational member. Organization cultures that are counterproductive are those which foster dependency, restrict personal autonomy, encourage dysfunctionality, and punish entrepreneurial spirit. These are cultures that fail to self-actualize (reference Maslow's hierarchy of needs).

Organization culture can be thought of as the context in which behaviors can be characterized and assessed. It is the environmental code that prompts people to act in certain ways to "fit in" at different levels and to perform in "expected" ways. For example, customers entering a fine dining establishment understand they are expected to dress appropriately, deport themselves in a dignified manner, wait to be seated at an assigned table, and ultimately, pay a premium price for the experience. Yet, there are usually no formal rules that are posted stating how guests are supposed to dress or how they are to behave. Once seated at their table with friends or other guests, they may adjust their behaviors to a more relaxed and interactive mode. This analogy equates to organizational cultures, wherein the overarching culture may prompt people to act one way; whereas, once they settle into their own departments or business units, their behavior may change somewhat from the corporate norm.

Bringing about change on an organizationwide basis requires considerable understanding on what is needed and why it is needed; it requires superior change-management ability and systems to realize targeted results. Elements of organization culture include how people work together; how responsible they feel for the success of the enterprise; how ethically they behave; how they interact with and respond to customers; how they think about the quality of the company's goods and services; how prideful they feel about the mission of the enterprise; and ultimately, how fulfilled people feel in having a say in the business or making a difference in people's lives as a result of the work they perform. In the end, highly constructive and productive cultures lead to optimum outcomes.

Up to 40% improvement in performance can be achieved by changing an organization's culture. According to Jeffery Pfeffer and Thomas D. Dee II, professor of organizational behavior, Graduate School of Business, Stanford University, providing training, status equalization, employment stability, and strong recognition and reward programs can propel any number of organizations to enviable levels of success. To remain viable and competitive, even service sector entities such as utilities, financial institutions, and government services, are recognizing the need to shift from transaction-based systems to ones that are more relationship focused, that is, compassionate. Such changes require enormous changes in organizational culture, as well as in supporting structures, that is, operational, technological, human resource systems, and policy structures. Because "structure follows strategy," it is virtually impossible to realize shifts in organizational culture unless changes in structure occur to support such seismic shifts.

Any number of technical systems have been developed over time to plan, facilitate, and gauge the degree to which change occurs. Such systems include: the Organizational Culture Inventory by Human Synergistics International (based in the United States); and Gallup's Clifton Strengths, formerly StrengthsFinder, with company locations in 30 regional city centers in North America. Such systems promote teamwork, employee engagement, organization change, and performance improvement. The systems developed by Human Synergistics enable organizations to improve organization cultures and, in turn, their leaders to be more constructive, achievement oriented, self-actualizing, and team oriented.

Similarly, proponents of Gallup's Clifton Strengths technology indicate that employees who are assessed and whose strengths are optimized utilizing Gallup's system are six times as likely to be engaged at work, 7.8% more productive in their role, three times as likely to have an excellent quality of life (work/life balance), and six times as likely to do what they do best every day.

For Herb Kelleher, founder of Southwest Airlines, it was important to create a culture of "love," "fun," and "outstanding customer service" (Kidadl, 2021). His vision jettisoned the airline to become one of the nation's most successful and admired companies. Beginning in 1971 Southwest grew to become the most popular and profitable airlines that today carries more than 120 million passengers a year. He eliminated onerous fees and unnecessary services and used less expensive secondary airports like Love Field in Dallas. He paid employees well, avoided layoffs and instilled a spirit of fun that resulted in increased customer loyalty. Herb Kelleher was a masterful artist and benevolent designer of a constructive organization culture. Today the organization employs more than 56,000 employees and topped more than 130 million passengers in 2019. Southwest coined "Transfarency" to describe its philosophy of treating customers honestly and fairly and keeping low fares low.

The goal for Novell Nouveau was to beat Microsoft at its own game. After rebuffing a takeover attempt by the giant corporation, Novell Nouveau went on an acquisition binge of its own. The strategy was to acquire a premier word processing company that could rival Microsoft and Microsoft's "Microsoft Word," in particular. So, in 1994 Raymond Noorda, chief executive officer (CEO) for then the second largest software company, acquired WordPerfect corporation for $1.4 billion in stock. Novell was to become a "software powerhouse," delivering "stand-alone, software suites, groupware, and network applications that were to define new capabilities for information systems," according to WordPerfect's leading executive. Two years later WordPerfect was sold for less than one seventh of its original purchase price. The reason for the failed strategy: "The cultures were very, very different," as reported by Novell's successor CEO, Robert Frankenberg (Clark, 1996).

Taking the role of the dominator, management of Novell Nouveau assumed their ways and methods to be superior to those of WordPerfect. They eliminated the sales force, assuming the Novell Nouveau organization could take over the sales and marketing function and went on to make a host of other mistakes. Indeed, their experience was similar to those of a majority of acquiring firms. Generally, 80% of acquisitions and mergers fail to perform to management's expectations, and the overarching factor in most instances is a failure to understand and manage organization culture.

Ethics and Values

Consider the various philosophical systems that are used to guide the values of an organization: *Teleology*, where the end justifies the means; *deontology*, where process is more important than the outcomes; *relativism*, where situational ethics prevail and one equivocates depending on what might "look good"; *virtue ethics*, where one is answering to a "higher calling"; and justice, a "by the book" approach. Each of these systems affect investor relations, customer relations, marketplace reputation, employee morale, business valuation, litigation, and whistle blowing. Compassion advocates must choose the approach that best speaks to the integrity of the organization and its individual members.

Shoshana Zuboff, coauthor of *The Support Economy: Why Corporations Are Failing Individuals and the Next Episode of Capitalism* (Zuboff & Maxmin, 2004), pointed to the abuses at WorldCom, Enron, and other organizations to affirm the view that any number of business organizations—and, I would add, some public institutions—are failing to honor the implicit and explicit commitments to key stakeholders, namely investors, customers, employees, and the community at-large. (Substitute taxpayers, citizens, government employees, and society in general, when it comes to the public sector.) The current model of capitalism and wealth creation is obsolete, she argued. But, from my perspective, before we throw the baby out with the bathwater, we need to strike at what I regard as the crux of the problem—leadership and a need for responsible *values* and *ethical behavior*.

Millions of pages have been written over the years about management and management practices. Yet, the "message" of doing the right thing apparently has not hit home with some. L. Dennis Koslowski, along with his chief financial officer, was accused of looting Tyco International of more than $600,000 in unapproved pay raises, bonuses and company loans. Charged with grand larceny, falsifying business records and violating state business laws, Koslowski was known to have squandered millions more of the company's money on inappropriate "business" and personal expenses. Martha Stewart may not have been charged with insider trading, but her guilty verdict for obstructing justice was enough to send her away, while her company and stockholders lost millions in the process.

Lost in all the theory and expert advice about "managers," "leaders," and "servant leaders" are the fundamental values of *doing the right thing*, *doing unto others as you would have them do unto you*, doing *good* in the world. Our system works best when people—at all levels of responsibility—act as *principled proponents of ethical values* and *stewards* of valued resources, be those resources be employees and their wages and benefit plans, stockholders and their investment savings, or the ecological gifts of clean air, safe water, and national reserves.

Returning to our story of Aaron Feuerstein, we see he was a man of values, believing in the worth of his employees, in the metaknowledge they had to perform virtually flawlessly in executing their responsibilities, and in the principle of doing the "right thing" for some greater good. He could easily have pocketed the insurance money on his loss, left the city to deal this the misfortune of losing a business and the unemployed, and packed for retirement. Instead, he did what he thought was the right thing to do for his employees, his community, and the economy. Feuerstein was a man of principles.

Today we are witnessing one of the greatest conflicts within American society with respect to values, specifically between truth/honesty, and the "big lie." We are seeing played out on a global stage the political conflict within a specific political party and between a former administration and the present administration. It is not for me to deal with this in this writing, but suffice it to say, Values matter, and the philosophical system by which these differences will be settled remains to be seen. In the meantime, the implications and ramifications with respect to workers and the workplace are enormous. The conflicts over values, policies, and politics affect wages, gender inequities, immigration, healthcare, systemic racism, LGBTQ issues, and more. The reverberations of such conflicts further exacerbate the condition of "anomy" within the workforce, as different factions compete, argue, and discriminate against one another, even though some organizations have attempted to ameliorate differences in the workforce by creating employee resource groups (ERGs). Furthermore, such reverberations are spilling out into the general populace in the form of hateful acts against Asian Americans and Pacific Islanders, Muslims, Jews, Mexicans, people of color, and other minorities. Now more than ever our society needs compassion and compassion advocates.

In the end, perhaps William Shakespeare's Polonius may have said it best when he stated, "This above *all*: to *thine own self* be *true*, and it *must follow*, *as* the *night* the *day*, *Thou* canst *not* then be false to *any man*" (Hamlet, Act 1, Scene 3). Certainly, there are those who march to their own drummer and are true to what they believe is right. In the clamor of everyday work life, people venture out to their places of employment or take their places at in-home workstations, setting aside their own life struggles to produce a product or provide some service to others. Like the hospice nurse who believes it is her mission to accompany the terminally ill on the final leg of their life journey, so her patients feel the caring and compassion of another human being. Like the copy center employee who loves to work with customers, while producing creative presentations that bring a sparkle to their eyes and the promise of favorable impressions with *their* customers. Like the exuberant airport baggage handler who leaps over the conveyor system and races to the transport truck to ensure your bags get to the plane on time, or like the dedicated teacher whose passion in life is to kindle a desire for learning in the hearts and minds of every student. Something at the core of their being motivates them to perform in a manner that puts the needs of those they serve above their own—and in so doing they are fulfilled in ways that are more satisfying and more rewarding than any anticipated fame or promise of reward.

What truly amazes me is that these "miraculous" deeds, these "heroic" acts continue to take place in the context of workplaces that brandish the threat of immanent termination in the form of employment-at-will policies and the routine downsizing of the corporate workforce. While loyalty between employers and employees is virtually dead and trust in leadership and institutions themselves continues to decline, somehow the flame of workplace 'heroism' continues to flicker and, in some quarters, blaze with startling brilliance.

Diversity and Inclusion

In a world replete with bigotry, anger, misogyny, fear of foreigners (xenophobia), and despair, the most effective antidote appears to be *compassion*. Globally, economic, social, and demographic trends are conflated in such a way as to ignite intergroup conflicts. For the organization focused on capitalizing on diversity, innovation, and resulting wealth, leadership must focus on the extent to which it can change an organization and the wide range of factors it must consider in order to achieve desired outcomes. It must adopt a broader vision of inclusion—one that focuses not only on the organization itself but also on the context in which it operates—locally, nationally, and globally.

Changing an organization from "diversity tolerant" and "respectful of diversity" to "totally inclusive" is critical in today's competitive marketplace, and it requires deliberate actions. The facts speak for themselves: increased diversity leads to increased innovation and ultimately to new wealth. Once again, analytics can determine how inclusive an organization is and how receptive it is to reap the rewards of innovation brought about by an amalgam of diverse opinions, experiences, and ideas. And again, we recommend the use of analytical tools that assess where an organization is and what actions need be taken to realize the wealth that is available to the entity.

Michàlle E. Mor Barak, posits that "changing the organization's culture from merely 'diversity tolerant' or 'respectful of diversity' to *truly inclusive* (must) be done through deliberate actions" at a systems level—within the work organization itself; through corporate-community collaborations; through state/nation collaborations; and through international collaborations (Mor Barak, 2017, p. 319.)

In the United States, building on his campaign promises, the 45th president issued various executive orders in 2017—from the so-called Muslim ban to the ban on transgender personnel serving in the military—which, while energizing his base, ignited bitter conflicts and a series of lawsuits and legal judgments blocking his edicts which various parties termed "discriminatory," "unconstitutional," and "anti-American." Federal agencies, like Immigration and Customs Enforcement and the FBI, as directed, pushed the limits of their authority to find and deport undocumented workers, the so-called "illegal aliens." Subsequently, the administration embarked on another strategy called "denaturalization," where the citizenship of immigrants was to be reevaluated to determine if some condition that might have existed before becoming a citizen would warrant revocation of citizenship and immediate deportation. Fortunately, much of these restrictive policies issued by executive order by "45" either have been or are being reversed. Yet, many of these same groups continue to be under attack by state legislatures.

Any number of bright spots are occurring in the workplace, however. In February of 2021, for example, Humana, Inc. announced that it received a score of 100 on the Human Rights Campaign Foundation's 2021 Corporate Equality Index, the nation's foremost benchmarking survey and report measuring corporate policies and practices related to LGBTQ workplace equality. Humana joins the ranks of 767 major U.S. businesses that also earned top marks in 2021. It was the eighth year in a row that Humana received the top score.

Celebrating diverse backgrounds and creating an environment of inclusion is at the heart of Humana's commitment to creating a work environment in which every associate can bring his or her whole being to work—no matter what the individual's background or ethnic makeup might be. One way that Humana does this is through its nine employee network resource groups (NRGs). NRGs provide personal, experience-based forums for exchanging ideas, building community, and driving measurable business outcomes in order to help the company see through a diverse lens. Each forum is associate led and associate driven. The seven NRGs include: Caregivers; HAPI—Asian/Pacific Islander; IMPACT—African American; Pride—LGBTQ and allies; SALUTE—Veterans; Unidos—Hispanic and Latino; and WNRG—Women. Beyond these NRGs, the company has additional groups that focus on disability, young professionals and new dads.

Enter the newest consideration in diversity management: *intersectionality*. Taking the concepts of diversity and inclusion to a higher level, senior consultant Wade Davis advocates the concept of "intersections of diversity" or intersectionality." A former National Football League player, he played for the Tennessee Titans, the Washington Redskins, and the Seattle Seahawks, as well as for two different teams within the National Football League Europe league. Davis is a thought leader, public speaker, and consultant on gender, race, and orientation equality. He is the National Football League's first LGBTQ inclusion consultant and currently consults for numerous professional sports leagues on issues at the intersection of sexism, racism and homophobia. Some of his other clients include Netflix, Google, and a number of smaller tech companies. He focuses on empowering employees throughout organizational systems, especially the marginalized, to optimize engagement and inclusion. The concept of intersectionality recognizes that an individual may have more than one diversity attribute. For example, an individual may be female, African American, a senior and LGBTQ.

It is important to note that some companies, such as Deloitte, are stepping away from ERGs, the equivalent to Humana's NRG's, and engaging a different approach, one they regard as a type of intersectionality. To include those unintentionally left out of the ERG's, such as White males, they are diverging away from separate categories such as age, veteran status, gender, et cetera. Instead, the company is forming "councils" comprised of a mixture of various employee types to focus on diversity issues. The company still claims to be committed to increasing women and minorities in its workforce, but their strategy reportedly is now one of what they regard as unification rather than separation. Their goal is for everyone to join in the effort by being valued as whole persons rather than individuals grouped according to separate classifications or types. At least, this is their premise.

Consultant Wade Davis has a different perspective on this approach. His conclusion is that Deloitte and a few others engaging in this approach are, in effect, recentering White males. They are trying to avoid risk. He contends there is no need to eliminate ERG's, but by moving in the direction of "intersectionality," organizations can find ways to bring White males into the conversation. People in these distinct groups or ERG's still need their "space" to vet their needs and their issues. Essentially, in large measure, Davis is advocating for a change in organization culture and the way in which people relate to one another, respect one another, and work with one another. Fundamentally, his premise is one of compassionate inclusion.

Compassion as a Currency

In his work *Punished by Rewards: The Trouble With Gold Stars, Incentive Plans, A's, Praise, and Other Bribes,* Alfie Kohn effectively demonstrates why contrivances and manipulation are less effective than respectful, thoughtful appreciation of people and the work they perform. Indeed, systems that engage employees respectfully and with compassion are far more effective. From our own research and experience we have found that people commit themselves to work that is meaningful and to organizations that appreciate them as whole human beings, rather than some unnecessary appendage that can be "distanced" or eliminated with the next round of budget cuts. The relationship becomes more intimate, more impactful not only with respect to the organization and its people but also between the organization and the ultimate customer. Indeed, compassion is a currency in and of itself.

The trouble with most reward systems is that they are, at a minimum, benign as to their effect and, more commonly, punishing. Yes, that's right. Punishing. And, for minimum wage jobs, the pay is blatantly punishing. So, what is the alternative? Well, consider the fact that people who work in many nonprofit organizations receive a fraction of what they would make in a comparable for-profit position, yet they are engaged in a way that they would not be otherwise. The answer: they are committed to the mission of the organization and the work they do is perceived as a "calling." They are making a difference in the lives of the people they serve. So, let's take a closer look at what I have coined the "Five Rs" (Bowen, 2006).

We begin with *responsibility*. Few organizations typically design "jobs" with the employee in mind. In fact, "job descriptions" usually look like extensive to-do lists with the catchall phrase at the end, "*and other tasks as directed by management*." The underlying message is, "Do whatever I tell you to do." Not a very inspiring message for today's workforce! And certainly not one that integrates well with an effective recognition and reward strategy. Designing jobs should be more about *profiling work processes* and *desired outcomes*, with employees involved as codesigners. Moreover, the work must be predicated on the principles of *respect* for the person doing the job and *appreciation* for how all parties can "add value" or "make a difference." Let's face it! Work is a creative process. It is an expression of *self.* No one really enjoys boring, repetitive, menial activity, especially not today's *free agent* worker. People generally want to feel that what they do adds value—whether providing a service or producing some tangible product. When work processes are designed collaboratively, responsibility is automatically built into the process. That is what *empowerment* is really all about, that is, having *accountability* and *responsibility*. Henry Ford was known for his straightforward approach to "partnering" with employees in designing jobs. He reportedly would take a difficult production job to the "laziest" (substitute "most resourceful") worker on the line to see how many shortcuts could be taken. To be sure, workers involved in this way felt valued and took full ownership for the production process once it hit their station. The efficiency of their redesign process resulted in improved profitability—saving both time and money.

Respect: Respect is one of the most critical dimensions of organizational life. Jeffrey Pfeffer, Stanford Graduate School of Business, maintains organizations with "pro-people practices" tend to perform up to 30 and 40% better over time (Pfeffer, 2018). Such organizations include Southwest Airlines, Men's Wearhouse, Toyota Motor Manufacturing, among others. Respectful organizations build cultures of continuous learning, teamwork, and genuine caring and concern for people—employees, customers, communities, suppliers, investors—indeed, all key stakeholders. Performance review systems are aimed at building confidence and competence, unlike other systems that are challenged to hold down raises and root out some percentage of the workforce regardless of their competitive value in the marketplace. "Please" and "thank you" are courtesies extended to organizational members and customers alike. Information—the lifeblood of every knowledgeable organization—flows freely throughout the system, as people are valued and respected for the intellectual capital they contribute. And, prudent risk-taking is encouraged in the interest of building *excellent* organizations. Furthermore, employees in such constructive organizations are respected and managed holistically. Feelings, ideas, and actions are valued and attended to. People are appreciated not only for what they know and do but also for the Emotional Intelligence they bring to the organization.

Relationships: Think back to your childhood school days and some of the teaching styles of your instructors. Remember the strict disciplinarian who taught by fear and intimidation? Not much focus on the 'joy of learning' with that teacher. Then there was the "feel good" teacher who pasted smiley faces and stars on your papers to encourage you to do your best and praise you when you did. According to Alfie Kohn (author of *Punished by Rewards*, 1993) that strategy *distracts* from the joy of both learning and working. On the other hand, the constructive strategy of an effective teacher focuses all attention on the process of discovery and personal development. Students are taught to think for themselves and to strive continuously for rewards of enlightenment and mastery. Similarly, the strategy of the effective leader is one of facilitation and education.

Doing *great* work builds competence and self-esteem, wins customers, and enhances organizational reputation as a whole. Because motivation is an *inside* job—something individuals chose to unleash under the right circumstances—the effective leader must focus on creating environments that are conducive to workers getting motivated. Coaching, teaching, supporting, guiding—all are strategies that have the best chance of producing the right outcomes. It is not easy, and you cannot "throw money" at the situation to make it happen. Leadership is an art, as much as a skill—one, I suspect, any number of middle managers did not have who were downsized over the last decade or so.

The quality of relationships with coemployees is equally important. Being part of a team, working with "great people," and having *fun*—that "spice" of creativity—enhances products and services. I know of any number of people in the workplace who love their jobs and the people they work with—including their management—who could make more money someplace else but who choose to stay with the team that hired them.

Recognition: It is not so much about getting credit as it is about being appreciated. Too many organizations waste valuable time, energy and resource on gestures of questionable value, such as, parking spaces for employees of the month, tickets for two at an upscale restaurant, et cetera. Sure, everyone is doing it. It may even be expected. But, what about recognition that comes in the form of assignments to join a special project or lead a study team or scope out a new system for the department or company? If the response in your organization to such invitations is, "Thanks; I'd love to!" then you're building the right kind of organization. If, on the other hand, it's "Pay me, and I'll do it!" then your department or company is far from reaching its full potential. Too much effort and money are spent in corporate America on building systems of extrinsic reward, that is, prizes, incentives contests, while not enough goes into creating intrinsic rewards, that is, genuine opportunities to contribute, become more knowledgeable, and develop professionally.

Understandably, recognition also comes in the form of promotions and public accolades. In organizations where the emphasis is on achieving as a team, internal politics and aggressive competition are appropriately low, while crediting others with a "job well done" is the standard. For any number of employees, particularly in entry level and minimum wage positions, the "psychic income" of being openly and regularly appreciated goes a long way toward enhancing worker retention and employee commitment.

Rewards: While Rewards are important, they are fifth in importance with respect to the 5 Rs. If people are paid fairly and competitively and they are informed as to how the system works, pay is a "satisfier," to quote Frederick Herzberg, but not a motivator. To provide optimum return on investment, however, rewards must be an integral part of an overall recognition and reward strategy—linking business goals and objectives with the other four (4) R's. Beginning with job profiles, rewards must be aligned with compensable factors centering on ***Responsibility***, *e.g.*, "satisfying customers," "building quality products," and, as an example for managers, "increasing workforce competence." Outcomes such as these can be quantified. Goals can be set that are mutually agreed upon by managers and employees. Job profiling also provides tools for hiring, training, and organization development. Other reward elements, such as ESOPs, 401(k)'s, and the like, should be clearly linked to company performance, and organizational members should receive periodic updates on how their efforts are impacting the bottom line.

Respect can be measured and compensable in terms of "building self-esteem," "enhancing company reputation," "exemplifying company values," et cetera. Effective relationships can be measured in terms of "teamwork," "strategic leadership," and "customer service." And both, intrinsic and extrinsic rewards can then be awarded and allocated for recognition purposes. Fundamental to the basic design of such systems in compassion.

Stewardship

When people and organizations join to serve the interests of others, they are giving credit to the concept of stewardship and by extension "enlightened self-interest." For example, when an organization chooses to support a segment of the population needing employment, that organization is helping that populace and themselves mutually. When a leader perceives that his or her role is to enhance the value of workers both for themselves and for the organization, that effort is an act of stewardship. To enhance the value and the reputation of an organization in the larger community, it is important to incorporate the concept and the actions of stewardship into one's portfolio of strategic initiatives.

Just as in our opening story of Aaron Feuerstein and Malden Mills, where Feuerstein perceived a commitment to his community, any number of organizations today recognize that a commitment of some sort to its larger community not only enhances the reputation of the organization but also the commitment of its workers. Younger job entrants in particular are attracted to organizations that are engaged in some sort of social responsibility.

Taken to the next level, some workplaces create an environment that is conducive to acts of selfless service, wherein employees are invited to respond, in a sense, to a higher calling. The South African expression, *Umuntu, Ngumuntu, Ngabantu* (pronounced: untu, muntu, abantu) loosely translated means "we are who we are through others." In other words, how we relate to and care about other people, defines the kind of person or people we are. For those who do good, by extension, the spiritual meaning is that: love is gracious; love is kind; it is a bond that cannot be broken; it is like a mighty flame that cannot be extinguished.

At the core of this belief is that we are a people of a larger universe and that our values are reflected in actions we take accordingly. Key stakeholders in any number of organizations today expect their people to engage in socially responsible endeavors. Servant leaders as described by Jim Collins (2005) play a critical role in creating, implementing, and sustaining socially responsible behaviors.

Where does one go to find out about stewardship? One might suggest connecting with a religious organization or people on some spiritual or humanitarian mission. One such person versed in the concept of stewardship is Deacon Lucio Caruso, former director of mission advancement for Catholic charities in the Archdiocese of Louisville. He asserts, "stewardship is about valuing precious resources—people, our planet, and all the gifts entrusted to us for safekeeping" (Bowen, 2020, p. 62). I believe we are responsible for protecting and enhancing the value of these resources for future generations and that we must leave these treasures and the world in which we live in better condition than when we arrived and assumed responsibility for them.

Volunteer Mary Sullivan, who has been actively engaged with Catholic Relief Services, expressed the concept of stewardship in this way,

> I think people who are committed to stewardship want to create a "legacy." They may never see the fruits of their labor, but somehow, they sense the good will be there at some point in the future. We, who work in this area of relief services, know we are building bridges for those who may not have hope but who need expectations for overcoming adversity, whether that adversity is poverty, a physical handicap, or emotional distress. And, when I sit 24 inches away from some young girl who is making progress in her life and who is modest about her story, she becomes my new hero. Yes, it's hard to change expectations, but that is my job. That is my mission. Changing expectations is stewardship. (Bowen, 2020, pp. 62–63)

Just as some view consumerism as the opposite of environmentalism, so too greed and selfishness can be viewed as the opposite of enlightened self-interest. According to Alexis de Tocqueville (Democracy in America, 1835), when people join together voluntarily to further the interests of the group by doing "right," they in turn are serving their own interests as well as the interests of others. One such organization advancing the notion of enlightened self-interest is United Parcel Service. It was at the office of Catholic Charities in Louisville that I found Larry Rosa, HR workforce planning supervisor, recruiting immigrant workers to help staff his packaging operations, while helping to lift these recruits out of poverty.

Compassion can come in all sizes, shapes, colors, and forms, he asserts. Something that is good for someone else can also be good for oneself. For Larry Rosa, the competency of "stewardship" truly comes in the form of enlightened self-interest. His "direct-to-the-point" explanation is that the stewardship program at United Parcel Service—called Global Gateways—is about helping others find a "gateway to the future." And it is actually one of several programs that are designed with enlightened self-interest in mind. According to Rosa,

> Global Gateways is about helping people achieve their dreams. It's about families finding hope. It's about people finding work. It's about the company achieving its objectives. I can't stress this enough. It's a winning situation for our people. It's a winning situation for the company. It's a winning situation for the community. It's a win-win situation for everyone. (Bowen, 2020, p. 64)

Leadership

Make no mistake. There have been many pages devoted over the years to the subject of leadership: like "Snakes in Suits" by Babiak and Hare (2006), "The Leadership Challenge" by Kouzes, and Parker (2017), and many, many more. Unfortunately, none capture the essence of compassionate leadership. Yet, compassionate leadership is what is needed now more than ever. One of the most effective things a leader can do is to complete a self-assessment profile that identifies the specific thinking and behavioral styles the leader thinks he or she exhibits. Then have feedback from at least twelve others on the styles they experience being exhibited by the leader. The summary of their feedback compared to the personal profile will pinpoint areas for improvement as well as areas to be emphasized.

If we were to envision an organization in the shape of a pyramid, we might hypothesize that the base represents workers with the most fundamental responsibilities, and the ascending tiers, workers with increasing levels of responsibility, and "management" at the top. Through organizational transformation the desired end state would be to invert the pyramid so that organizational members are at the top and the empowering, compassionate leader on point at the base. While leadership is only one of our seven competencies of compassion, it is perhaps one of the most critical elements.

A leader's job is tougher today, because "followers" are understandably skeptical. Consequently, we all need to rededicate ourselves to being stewards of our resources—inspiring commitment, protecting the environment, garnering respect, and adding value to what we do. So, here's a list of seven attributes that I have found to be essential for responsible leadership:

- **Values-Centered:** Leaders do the right thing—even when confronted with the most difficult of choices. They do not dissemble, hide, or make excuses. They earn respect and inspire others to emulate their example.
- **Selfless:** Like rescue workers at a disaster scene, they focus on the welfare of others—safeguarding the human, tangible and financial resources for which they are responsible. (Aaron Feuerstein kept workers on payroll for months after Malden Mills was destroyed by fire, keeping his workforce available and committed for a magnificent recovery.)
- **Purposeful**—Leaders believe their lives have value and are intended for some useful purpose. Beyond goals and objectives, their vision is one of living and serving in ways that bring honor and meaning to themselves and those they serve.
- **Accountable**—Leaders empower themselves to take responsibility. Like President Truman, whose mantra was "The buck stops here," they take action in matters that matter most and intervene wherever they see injustice or the need to make a difference.
- **Integral**—They believe they are part of some larger whole—being *integrated* with a sort of world community. At the same time, they experience a quiet *integrity* of values, purpose, and accountability that occurs frequently below the level of their own awareness.
- **Disciplined**—Instilled in every leader is the 'muscle memory' to stay the course—doing the right thing, leading by example, and encouraging the best in others.
- **Courageous**—And, finally, they find the wherewithal to avoid the temptation of greed and avarice. The basis for our capitalistic system is to provide for the common good with products and services that benefit all. Leaders perform as stewards and have courage to recognize serving is *not* about them. It is about others.

Mary Kay Ash, the late founder of Mary Kay Cosmetics, built one of the largest direct-sales cosmetics companies in the world. Her vision was to enhance the self-esteem of women by providing the means to their achieving financial independence. May Kay Ash was an exceptional leader but a quintessential steward as well. Steve Jobs, who built the Apple corporation, was indeed brilliant, but he was a terrible CEO according to Leander Kahney (2019), who has spent much of his writing career covering Apple. Jobs was successful because he kept hiring people who were better at leading that he was, people like the current Apple CEO Tim Cook. A brilliant executive, as well, Cook is actually a better CEO than Jobs ever was according to Kahney.

Corporate Social Responsibility

It should be noted that millennials especially are committed to organizations that have corporate social responsibilities policies. Upwards of 76% of these job seekers today actually look for companies with corporate social responsibility programs, yet only 47% of U.S. organizations have such policies at this time. Needless to say, for the organization of the future, having corporate social responsibilities policies provides a competitive edge in recruitment and a sustaining advantage in lowering turnover and increasing retention.

For Semonin Realtors, a Berkshire Hathaway Affiliate located in Louisville, Kentucky, social responsibility comes from the heart—from the heart of the people who are engaged in good deeds ... from the heart of the organization that is called to a higher purpose. As Stacy Durbin, general manager with Semonin Realtors expressed, social responsibility exhibited as works of kindness and caring is "good for the soul" (Bowen, 2020, pp. 86–87). Moreover, it translates to the bottom line in reputation, performance, and profit. One such endeavor for Semonin Realtors is Habitat for Humanity. Stacey's firm is one of the largest and most respected real estate companies in Kentucky with approximately 470 agents. Semonin's connection with Habitat represents the "perfect partnership" according to Stacy. "We are about achieving home ownership for people, and with Habitat it is about achieving home ownership for people who might not have the ability to own a home through traditional means such as with mortgage lending." So, what about Semonin's agents, employees, and contractors? Stacy again, "Everyone comes to work for different reasons, be it financial, social, philosophical, or because it is something they are passionate about or feel driven to do. With Semonin there is a unique opportunity to engage in something extra, something that feels meaningful and larger, in the sense of compassion in action. Seeing the joy of a little girl who is going to have her own bedroom or the tears on the face of a grateful mother who is going to have some stability in her life with a roof over her head is just indescribable.

Stacy Durbin serves on the local board for Habitat and is committed to making a difference in the world. As for the benefit to the company, well the bottom-line impact is inestimable. Employee retention is high. The esteem of the workforce is strong. The reputation of the firm is enhanced, and the contribution to the community is priceless. Stacy Durbin and Semonin Realtors believe in and are passionate about the competency of corporate social responsibility.

PUTTING IT ALL TOGETHER

The seven key competencies of compassion identified in this narrative: values, leadership, stewardship, service, recognition, culture, and diversity, when implemented strategically, comprise the "new-age currency" that drives success (see Figure 5.1). Indeed, the return on investment is realized in improved employee engagement and retention; optimal organizational performance; and increased profit up to 40% and more. Now more than ever organizations will need to become compassion driven. The pandemic has taken its toll. We are witnessing a transformation of the

Figure 5.1

The Seven Key Competencies of Compassion

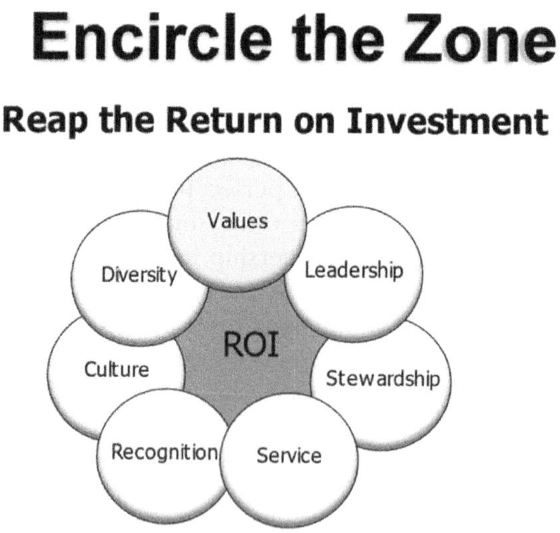

Source: ©2021 Building Better Worlds of Work, LLC.
All rights reserved.

traditional "office" and "factory," as organizations race to reduce square footage and shrink corporate overhead. "Working remotely" is becoming more acceptable today and, indeed, more desirable from the perspective of both employer and employee. Any number of workers are opting *not* to return to the job site, preferring instead to work from home. Technology may provide the bridge for communication and production, yet "organizational distancing" is contributing to poor communication, loss of "team spirit," and increased turnover. Future success will require management to become masterful in monetizing compassion in many ways and in many forms. For example, communications will need to be optimized to inspire employee engagement and improve performance. Recognition and reward systems will need to be designed with the employee and compassion in mind. Stewardship and corporate social responsibility initiatives will need to be ingrained in the compassion fabric of organizations if they are to enhance their branding, improve their market reputation, and ultimately ensure their success. Monetizing compassion will require strategic integration of the competencies of compassion described earlier to achieve optimum results and return on investment.

For compassion to become the new-age currency, organizational leaders and professionals will need to become compassion advocates. So, come on board and become an agent of change wherever you land. Your "worlds" and the worlds around you will thank you.

REFERENCES

Babiak, P., & Hare, R. D. (2006). *Snakes in suits*. Harper.

Bowen, R. B. (2006). Practice the five R's to motivate people. *HR Magazine: Guide to Managing People*, pp. 59–64.

Bowen, R. B. (2020). *Engaging the heart for people, performance, and profit: Seven competencies of compassion@work*. Building Better Worlds of Work® Press.

Collins, J. (2005). *Good to great and the social sectors: Why business thinking is not the answer*. HarperCollins.

Clark, D. (1996). Worst 10-year performer Novell. *The Wall Street Journal*.

Durkheim, E. (2006). *On suicide*. Penguin Books. (Original work published 1897)

Feuerstein, A. (n.d.). *AZQuotes.com*. https://www.azquotes.com/quote/1237122

Kahney, L. (2019). *Tim Cook: The genius who took Apple to the next level*. Portfolio/Penguin.

Kidadl. (2021, November 4). *Herb Kelleher quotes on inspiration*.

Kohn, A. (1993). *Punished by rewards: The trouble with gold stars, incentive plans, A's, praise, and other bribes*. Houghton Mifflin.

Kouzes, J., & Parker, B. (2017). *The leadership challenge*. Wiley.

Mor Barak, M. E. (2017). *Managing diversity* (4th ed.). SAGE.

Pfeffer, J. (2018). *Dying for a paycheck: How modern management harms employee health and company performance and what we can do about it*. HarperCollins.

Zuboff, S., & Maxmin, J. (2004). *The support economy: Why corporations are failing individuals and the next episode of capitalism*. Penguin.

CHAPTER 6

FROM DISRUPTION TO CONNECTION

How Mindful Conflict Management Builds Bridges During the Pandemic and Beyond

LaVena Wilkin

Even in the best of times, workplace conflicts can disrupt relationships, hinder productivity, and leave us feeling anxious about our leadership abilities. Most of us have learned that conflict is negative and needs to be either passively avoided or aggressively confronted so that we can put it behind us and move on. In fact, when people think of conflict, words such as fight, argument, struggle, and antagonism come to mind. Who wants to invite that negativity into their life? As a result, it is not surprising that many leaders avoid engaging in conflict situations. They may tell their employees to "go work it out," or they may ignore the situation altogether hoping it will simply go away (Wilkin, 2020a).

Rarely are either of these alternatives productive, and in fact, they are likely to exacerbate the situation and persistently create angst among employees and disrupt the workplace. In addition to the negative connotation of conflict, leaders often have not been trained in conflict manage-

Back to a New Normal: In Search of Stability in an Era of Pandemic Disruption—Insight From Practitioners and Academics, pp. 85–95

ment, so they simply respond as they learned in their families of origin: fight or flight. Again, these responses may escalate the conflict and allow it to spiral into destructive behaviors and outcomes.

Conflict management is difficult enough when individuals and teams are meeting face to face in the "normal" operation of business. Sitting across the table from someone provides a connection that may be missing when we are sitting in our home offices and interacting via a computer screen. As a result of working from home during the pandemic, employees not only feel disconnected from one another, but they are also dealing with other life stresses, such as homeschooling their children, economic fears, and health and safety concerns. Moreover, while conflicts still exist in a virtual environment, they can be more difficult for leaders to address and manage when face-to-face interactions are impossible and other distractions and fears influence employees' emotions and perspectives.

Forward-thinking leaders can help build bridges for employees that create a psychologically safe place for resolving the inevitable conflicts. In part, leaders make these connections when they become more mindful of themselves, their employees' needs, and the overall working environment. In addition, honing their communication skills and embracing emotional intelligence may help leaders skillfully maneuver through conflicts during times of emergencies, such as the pandemic, and beyond.

CONSTRUCTING A MINDFULNESS CONSCIOUSNESS

Mindfulness is sometimes perceived as a nebulous or new age concept that has nothing to do with the workplace. However, mindfulness is a valuable tool for helping leaders resolve conflicts and make better decisions (Riskin & Wohl, 2015; Yu & Zellmer-Bruhn, 2018). Mindfulness is defined as bringing attention and awareness to current experiences without judgment or attachment to an outcome (Brown et al., 2007). In today's work environment, where busyness, multitasking, and virtual meetings are normal ways of being, it can be difficult for leaders to focus their attention on what is happening in the moment. Additionally, when conflicts arise, it is easy to slip into mindlessness, act on autopilot, and revert to our comfort zones of fight or flight.

Practicing mindfulness provides stability and control over the conflict, and it encourages more positive emotional responses; therefore, we are less likely to respond negatively to the event. Mindfulness helps us understand and be more compassionate toward others, gain insights about ourselves, recognize we are all interconnected, and enables us to let go of habitual ways of thinking and acting (Riskin & Wahl, 2015). As a result, conflicts are less likely to escalate and lead to unproductive outcomes (Yu & Zellmer-Bruhn, 2018).

BEING MINDFUL THAT CONFLICT IS AN OPPORTUNITY

One of the first steps on the path to constructive conflict management is a mindful paradigm shift from believing conflict is something to either be avoided at all costs or aggressively confronted. Conflicts are a naturally occurring phenomenon within any organization. A somewhat surprising thought is that conflict is not negative. We all have conflicts, and in an organization, they can be essential for growth and progress. Conflict is a simply a symptom that something is not working, either a relationship or a process, and it is an opportunity to make necessary changes. The way we manage conflicts leads to either productive or unproductive outcomes (Wilkin, 2020a).

Avoiding the conflict or forcing an outcome can damage relationships, cause unnecessary disruptions in productivity, and it simply does not resolve the issue. On the other hand, employees are more likely to be on the same page, work toward common goals, and fulfill the organization's vision and mission when conflicts are effectively addressed. Managing conflicts constructively can strengthen relationships, provide insights into different points of view, and build bridges that connect us to more productive ways of doing business. Many leaders do not have effective conflict management skills because they have not been taught how to engage in these situations. The good news is that if we are not content with the outcomes of our conflict situations, there are steps we can take to improve them by developing and honing our abilities.

MINDFULLY BUILDING A PSYCHOLOGICALLY SAFE WORKPLACE

One of the first steps is to build a psychologically safe workplace. It is likely that people will not be open to engaging in constructive conflict management processes if they believe that sharing their problems will result in reprimands or other negative consequences. As a result, creating a psychologically safe workplace is critical for productive conflict management. Psychological safety, defined as an individual's perception that they will not be punished or embarrassed for speaking up with ideas, questions, concerns, or mistakes (Edmondson, 1999) was a challenging task prepandemic. Simply stated, the pandemic changed the way people lead and work as more and more of us began working from home. Consequently, it can be difficult to build a psychologically safe workplace when people are conducting business virtually and maneuvering through the personal issues that come with the concerns of basic needs, including physical safety.

Previously, separating work-related matters from personal issues was an unspoken rule, and many leaders made a concerted effort to avoid discussing private problems such as childcare or an individual employee's anxiety about health. Moreover, leaders never asked if their employees were sharing workspaces with spouses and children. It simply was not the leader's problem. However, sharing this space has added another level of concern regarding privacy and productivity. Working from home requires employees and leaders to have open and honest conversations about these matters and how they impact the way work completed.

Edmondson and Mortenson (2021) offer guidance for leaders to begin these conversations and create a culture of psychological safety as they navigate the unchartered territory created by the pandemic. The first step is to set the stage by beginning the conversation and recognizing that getting the work done is a shared problem which requires input from everyone to develop creative ways of doing business and assure customers are served, missions are accomplished, and responsibilities are met.

Leaders who are candid, humble, and vulnerable lead by example, and their employees are more apt to share their own concerns. Mutual sharing may take some time because employees may not initially feel safe, or they may not trust that what they say will not be used against them in some way. However, leaders who are mindful about their responses to shared information, who model respect for their employees, and who are genuine and honest (even when they make mistakes) can begin to build a psychologically safe workplace (Edmonson & Mortenson, 2021).

MAKING CONNECTIONS THROUGH MINDFUL COMMUNICATION

As we consider building the bridge of psychological safety that leads to constructive conflict management, communication skills, both listening and speaking. are the pillars for success. Communication provides the human connection everyone needs to feel respected and valued. Page et al. (2019) found that honest and considerate communication creates an environment of trust and respect. Without trust, employees are less likely to openly share concerns and problems, and it becomes easier to ignore conflicts. However, ignoring them does not make them go away. Instead, the conflicts fester, grow, and eventually they must be addressed.

Communication sounds like such an easy skill to acquire. The reality is that even in "normal" times it is difficult to master. One benefit in face-to-face encounters, is that we hear the spoken words and can intuit the feel-

Figure 6.1

The Essence of Listening

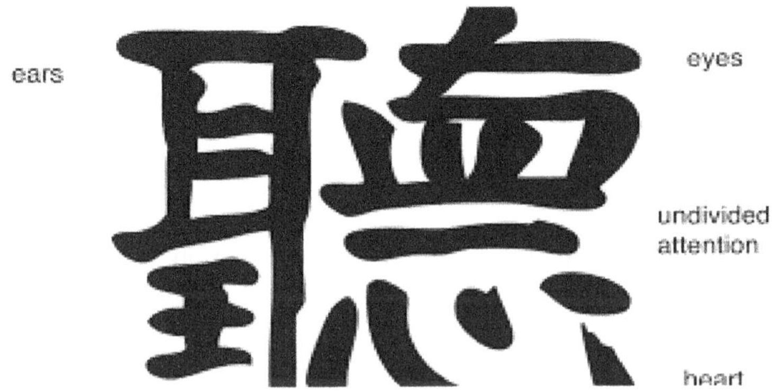

ings behind them. In addition, we observe the subtle nonverbal cues in those in-person meetings. However, communication problems have been exacerbated during the pandemic when much of our communication is via virtual meetings or written emails where we can misread tone and we lose the opportunity to watch for body language and other nonverbal cues.

Moreover, many approach listening from the perspective of taking turns talking. When the other person is speaking, instead of being fully engaged in conversation, we are thinking about how we will respond to them. As a result, we miss out on the essence of the message, and we lose the opportunity to inspire trust and build the human connection (Wilkin, 2020a). A more effective approach is to mindfully listen to understand, which requires us to pay careful attention to the message and the feelings of others. People often approach conversations from their own frame of reference. Acknowledge that their perceptions are valuable and let them know that you want to resolve the conflict.

The symbol in Figure 6.1 embodies the essence of listening. It symbolizes physical listening with our ears; being aware of nonverbal body language by watching for these cues; giving the person our undivided attention; and being fully present and engaged with our heart.

Mindful listening is a powerful tool that creates interconnectedness and promotes positive conflict management. Fortunately, it is a skill we can hone when we have an open mind and are willing to learn and practice.

An easy acronym for helping us improve our listening skills is REFLECT (Wilkin, 2020b):

R = Refrain from judging the speaker's ideas, words, or message
E = Empathize with the speakers by viewing the world through their lens
F = Focus your attention on the speaker watching for body language and other nonverbal cues
L = Listen to understand, not simply to respond
E = Engage in the conversation by asking open-ended questions
C = Clarify what you heard
T = Thank the speaker

Listening is one side of the communication equation. We must also pay close attention to how we deliver our message. People are not mind readers, so we need to be direct, yet polite. Use "I" statements that empower you and give you ownership of your own thoughts and feelings. Finally, when delivering your message, stay in the present and focus on the future outcomes. Reminding the other person of past mistakes can lead to resistance, and when the defensive walls go up, it is more difficult to resolve conflicts.

Being mindful of how we communicate and practicing open, honest, respectful communication where we suspend judgment and listen to the other person's viewpoints helps us learn about their values, needs, and expectations. As a result, we can discover their motivations and get to the root cause of the conflict and knowing what motivates others allows us to move toward productively managing the conflict.

BUILDING RELATIONSHIPS THROUGH EMOTIONAL INTELLIGENCE

No doubt, the pandemic brought a myriad of emotions and emotional responses to the forefront of workplace interactions. Fear, sadness, anger, and uncertainty have been the daily companions for some employees as they maneuvered a new way of accomplishing their professional goals while balancing their personal responsibilities. Emotions are the windows to people's inner core, and every conflict is connected to some emotion. If we did not care about the situation, there would not be a conflict, and emotions provide leaders with information that words alone do not offer. Becoming more mindful of emotions is one way to move from disruption to connection. Now more than ever, emotional intelligence reinforces conflict management; being mindful of this concept helps us transform conflicts into productive outcomes.

Unfortunately, even when people know the importance of managing conflicts productively, they often get caught up in the moment and fail to apply what they know. Riskin and Wahl (2015) attribute this to the "six obstacles" (p. 123) that create a lack of awareness or a lack of mindfulness. These include:

- excessively self-centered viewpoints.
- strong negative emotions.
- automatic, habitual ways of thinking, feeling, and behaving.
- sensitivity to emotions.
- insufficient social skills; and
- inadequate focus.

Goleman's (2005) model of five concepts of emotional intelligence addresses each of these obstacles. Although the six are presented as separate concepts, they are interconnected. For example, it is difficult to be self-regulated and motivated if you are not self-aware. Likewise, empathy for others is difficult if you are not aware of your own emotions and what triggers them (Wilkinson, 2019). Empathetic people develop and manage good relationships with others, which is also a part of the concept of social skills.

Self-awareness and self-regulation underpin emotional intelligence. Self-awareness is the ability to understand your own emotions and determine why you feel this way. Leaders who are self-aware listen to their emotions, but do not make decisions solely based on how they feel. They truthfully assess their strengths and weaknesses and continually strive to grow, develop, and learn more effective ways to interact with others. Self-regulation, the second component of emotional intelligence, is the ability to monitor; emotionally intelligent leaders do not allow others to push their hot buttons. When dealing with conflicts emotionally intelligent leaders are thoughtful, act with integrity, and adapt to necessary changes. Given these traits, it is easy to see how the attributes of self-awareness and self-regulation bolster psychological safety and improve mindful communication.

In addition, emotionally intelligent leaders are motivated to accomplish goals. They approach situations with optimism, and even if they are not successful, they tend to ask, "What is the lesson here?". They are mindful of the root cause of the problem, and they are aware of the positive opportunities associated with conflict.

Empathy is a one of the most critical concepts of emotional intelligence. In fact, Wilkinson (2019) says empathy is the glue that holds society together. It is the channel that connects people and provides a view of the world through the other person's lens. Empathy allows us to understand others' feelings and emotions (Wilkin, 2020a). Empathetic people are open and honest, and as a result, they easily cultivate relationships.

Through self-reflection and self-awareness, empathetic people create and live life authentically without being too quick to judge or stereotype others.

The final concept of Goleman's model (2005), social skills, encompasses the other four concepts. People with good social skills are team players, and they enjoy mentoring others and helping them grow within the organization. They understand that an organization is most successful when people play well together and communicating and building relationships are key factors in the way they interact with others.

BUILDING THE BRIDGE FROM DISRUPTION TO CONNECTION

While the constructs of psychological safety, communication, and emotional intelligence are always important considerations for leaders, the pandemic shone a spotlight on the criticality of becoming more mindful of each of them during turbulent periods. How do leaders develop mindfulness, especially when they are working to navigate the murky waters of the unknown themselves, accomplish their responsibilities, and inspire and motivate their employees? How do they overcome the six obstacles that can make it difficult to productively manage conflicts during stormy times?

Interestingly, publications ranging from blogs (mindful.org) to scholarly literature (Harvard Negotiation Law Review) advocate meditation as a powerful tool for developing mindfulness. Practicing meditation allows us to slow down, focus on what is important in the moment, self-reflect, and shift our thinking. While there is not one "right" way to meditate, Riskin and Wahl (2015) advocate sitting for a few quiet moments and simply concentrating on your breath, body sensations, emotions, and thoughts.

In addition, Riskin and Wahl's (2015) STOP tool can be used to create mindfulness quickly and help us focus on what is important in the moment. STOP is:

S = Stop what you are doing

T = Take a breath

O = Observe body sensations, emotions, and thoughts

P = Proceed with whatever you were doing

Developing mindfulness takes practice. However, when we can live in the moment, we can begin to appreciate others' contributions, we practice compassion, and we lead by example. As a result, we more effectively address and overcome the six obstacles that may be preventing us from productively managing conflicts.

MOVING FROM THEORY TO PRACTICE—A BRIEF CASE STUDY

Lily leads a team of financial advisors, and she and her employees began working from home when the pandemic brought the business world to a screeching halt. Working virtually, leading from home, and assuring the clients' needs are served has been challenging for her, and she has been looking forward to all her employees returning to the office. Finally, one by one, her team is coming back. However, Sam is not ready to return. His wife and son have health-related challenges, and he is not convinced that it is safe to be around others for eight to ten hours a day. He has protected himself and his family for the past year, and he does not want to lift the precautions now. Sam has two choices: to talk to Lily about his situation or to find another firm that would allow him to continue working from home for a while longer.

Fortunately, he feels comfortable having a candid conversation with Lily because she has demonstrated compassion toward her employees. She has taken great care to create a psychologically safe workplace, and she encourages her team to share their concerns without fear of retribution. Even under the most stressful situations, she listens to her team, is even-tempered, and makes informed decisions after listening to all the information. Sharing his home office with his wife and home schooling his son has not negatively impacted his productivity. In fact, he was the team's top performer last year. He does not want any special treatment, and he does not know how his teammates feel about returning to the office. However, Sam knows that he is not yet ready, and the thought of it makes him fearful. He asks Lily for a meeting to discuss his options.

Lily prides herself on her ability to motivate her team, and as a result, she has one of the most successful teams at the firm. However, it was not always this way. When Lily was first promoted to a leadership position, she was concerned about how her boss and her team would accept her. She did not encourage her team members to talk with her, and when mistakes were made, she was quick to blame the other person. When conflicts between team members occurred, she told the conflicted employees to figure it out. After all, they were adults who should be able to get along. By the end of each workday, she was so stressed that after a few months, she questioned whether she wanted to even stay at the firm. She realized that she was her own worst enemy, and if she did not make some changes to her approach, her negative thoughts would become a self-fulfilling prophecy.

Lily's first step to changing her leadership approach was to consciously think about her responses and reactions to conflict situations and to the people involved. She paid careful attention to her own emotions and why she felt this way. Many times, she reacted out of fear that others would see her as incompetent. As she became more self-aware, she was able to practice being calm, even in turbulent times. Interestingly, her calm approach encouraged her employees to trust her and talk more candidly about their challenges and their triumphs. Lily started listening to understand what her employees were saying, and she developed empathy for them. She realized they had good ideas that would improve the department's processes. Lily was no longer insecure in her abilities to lead her team or to help them resolve the inevitable conflicts that arise when people work together. When she feels anxious about a situation, she stops for a minute, identifies her emotions, takes a breath, and moves forward. The simple act of living in the present has helped her become a more effective manager, especially during the pandemic when her employees were stressed about how their life situations impacted their professional lives.

As a result, when Sam talked to her about his situation, she simply listened to his concerns. Even though she was eager to have the team together physically in one office space, she empathized with his situation. He was one of her top performers, and she did not want to lose him. Working together on a solution, they decided that he would continue to work from home for the next month, and then, they would reevaluate the future. Sam felt his needs were honored and respected, and Lily retained a valued employee.

CONCLUSION

The pandemic has provided an opportunity for leaders to reflect on conflict management processes within their organizations and to make any necessary changes that will help them productively resolve conflicts. If you slip into the mindset that conflict is negative, shift your thinking and remember that it is simply a symptom of something that needs changed, and this is the opportunity to make those changes. Psychologically safe workplaces begin with honest and respectful conversations that suspend judgment. Model the trust and openness you wish to create in the workplace, including listening to understand and suspending judgment. Be aware of your emotional responses and the emotional responses of others and ask, "What am I to learn from this?" The golden thread running through each of these interconnected concepts is mindfulness. To practice mindfulness, stop for a minute, focus on the present, and reflect on what is important in this moment. Be aware of your thoughts and your emotions. And just breathe.

REFERENCES

Brown, K. W., Ryan, R. M., & Creswell, J. D. (2007). Mindfulness: Theoretical foundations and evidence for its salutary effects. *Psychological Inquiry, 18*(4), 211–237. https://doi.org/10.1080/10478400701598298

Goleman, D. (2005). *Emotional intelligence: Why it can matter more than IQ*. Bantom Books

Edmondson, A. (1999). Psychological safety and learning behavior in work teams. *Administrative Science Quarterly, 44*, 350–383. https://doi.org/10.2307/2666999

Edmonson, A., & Mortenson, M. (2021). What psychological safety looks like in a hybrid workplace. *Harvard Business Review Digital Articles*, 1–7.

Page, L., Boysen, S., & Arya, T. (2019). Creating a culture that thrives. Fostering respect, trust, and psychological safety in the workplace. *Organizational Development Review, 51*(1), 28–35.

Riskin, L. L., & Wahl, R. (2015). Mindfulness in the heat of conflict: Taking STOCK. *Harvard Negotiation Law Review, 20,* 121–155. https://ssrn.com/abstract=2754646

Yu, L., & Zellmer-Bruhn, M. (2018). Introducing team mindfulness and considering its Safeguard role against conflict transformation and social undermining. *Academy of Management Journal, 61*(1), 324–347. https://doi-org.suscorp.idm.oclc.org/10.5465/amj.2016.0094

Wilkin, L. (2020a). From discord to harmony: Five skills for keeping your workplace humming. In L. Wilkin & T. Belak (Eds.), *From discord to harmony: Making your workplace hum* (pp. 319–332). Information Age.

Wilkin, L. (2020b). *Communication and conflict management.* CITI Program. https://www.citiprogram.org/members/index.cfm?pageID=125#view

Wilkinson, I. G. (2019). In praise of empathy: The glue that holds caring communities together in a fractured world. *Canadian Journal of Family and Youth, 11*(1), 234–291.

CHAPTER 7

BIG PROBLEMS, BIG DATA

The Critical Role of IT During an Era of Pandemic Disruption

Michael Hart

OVERVIEW

The harrowing effects of COVID-19 provides a daily reminder of the frailty of life. As COVID-19 reached epidemic levels throughout the world, information technology (IT) professionals worked diligently to support medical experts to inform people, prevent its spread, identify better treatments, and find long-term cures. Big data software and systems stepped up to the plate, providing IT infrastructure and services to support the mammoth pandemic response. Medical experts throughout the world have acted tirelessly to help treat patients but also identify how to prevent deaths and find effective vaccinations. Behind the scenes, IT professionals are supplying the medical community with the computing resources necessary to fulfill their roles more proficiently. In this chapter, we will outline examples of how IT is supporting healthcare amidst the pandemic but also its ability to support future demands during catastrophic events.

Back to a New Normal: In Search of Stability in an Era of Pandemic Disruption—Insight From Practitioners and Academics, pp. 97–110

BIG DATA SYSTEMS, IOT, AND INFORMATION SECURITY

Big data systems provide the platform necessary for medical professionals and researchers to carry out the fight against big pandemics (ElDahshan et al., 2020). Three emerging technologies with close interconnections are the internet of things (IoT), big data (BD), and information security (S). The latter three concepts coin the acronym "IoTBDS." IoT allows countless sensors to communicate across computer networks, facilitating the interaction and data collection of electronic devices ranging from vehicles to home electronics. Big data is derived from several "V's" including but not limited to data volume, velocity, variety, veracity, and value. Pivotal to the transportation and storage of data is information security. Big data loses its value without data privacy, secure data storage, and secure communication of network packets between devices (Chang et al., 2020). Together, these concepts facilitate the capabilities to store and analyze massive quantities of data, a substantial need during pandemics.

The COVID-19 pandemic has placed an even greater emphasis on IoTBDS to support eHealth and mHealth. At the heart of IoT are wireless sensor networks (WSNs) made up of numerous wireless connected devices. WSN connected devices can be self-configured with ease to monitor innumerable environmental parameters such as heartbeat, motion, sound, temperature, and/or pollution. Termed as "smart," IoT objects with WSN-based sensors are able to be controlled in mass remotely. Although WSNs have broad support for various medical applications, they are also advancing to meet specific healthcare needs. For instance, both eHealth and mHealth are able to leverage wireless body sensor networks (WBSNs) to monitor key human attributes specific to the contagious disease such as oxygen levels, respiration rate, electrocardiogram, and blood pressure (Li et al., 2021).

These sensor networks will only expand moving forward. In the future, WBSNs and several variations will allow medical experts to monitor patients from afar. Furthermore, artificial intelligence (AI) will enable computing devices to sense and respond to unique characteristics of different human systems. While one human being may have a high medical risk with a temperature of 102-degree Fahrenheit, another this may be 104 degrees. AI will be able to alert healthcare professionals of these differences with little to no human intervention.

Despite the latter innovations, the computer and data science communities have monumental tasks ahead to better support the healthcare community. More accurate sensors are needed to differentiate key symptoms between diseases. When appropriate data is available, machine learning is capable of finding patterns in the human body quickly, determining which drugs result in the greatest chance of survival in intensive care units, and providing more combinatory cross-lab results from experimental data. Even simple applications are within reach today that need additional exploration. Suppose that human taste sensors are connected through mobile IoT apps. Accurate analysis of the coinciding data collected could differentiate between COVID-19 and flu related symptoms.

Using the power of IoTBDS, a much stronger global response to novel diseases is possible. Rapid spreading pandemics like COVID-19 require a more united and coordinated effort from world leaders to collect, store, and secure relevant data to reduce the loss of human life. As international standards and policies mature, the computer and data science communities have begun building a foundation capable of improving a vast array of life saving capabilities. Regardless, it must continue to develop more proficient methods to collect accurate data, ensure data privacy, secure data, and share the results of data in forms easily consumable by all stakeholders. As wise stewards of vast quantities of data that leads to wisdom, data scientists also have a tremendous responsibility to present knowledge in forms that are not easily misinterpreted by individuals extrinsic to their discipline.

DATA VISUALIZATION AND MODELING

A prominent "V" of big data that is not always included in early big data frameworks is data visualization. Data must be given context, connotation, and comprehension, leading to insight and wisdom. In healthcare, data visualization and modeling have become paramount for individuals to effectively identify their levels of therapeutic risk and make informed decisions based upon these risks. As an example, the Coronavirus Resource Center at Johns Hopkins University (JHU) models critical trends in data, such as sequencing the DNA of SARS-CoV-2. These developments help researchers identify existing and mutating properties of the virus, such as whether new versions are more resistant to current vaccines or are more contagious. Central to the JHU center's recent popularity is a widely used COVID-19 dashboard that visualizes complex information pertaining to the pandemic.

On January 22, 2020, Dr. Lauren Gardner from the Department of Civil and Systems Engineering at Johns Hopkins University School of Engineering led efforts to launch the COVID-19 Dashboard. Figure 7.1 illustrates the interactive dashboard on May 17, 2021. The intuitive visualization tool allows users to filter data using parameters like the number of COVID-19 cases by country, region, state, and county. Users can zoom into a specific county in the United States and see localized data such as the number of cases and deaths. The dashboard, which Dr. Gardner credits PhD students Frank Dong and Hongru Du for helping create, has logged nearly 3 billion page views at the time of this writing (Faculty Lauren Gardner, n.d.). Dr. Gardner, along with other experts, focuses on virus diffusion by engineering dynamic models that not only shows prior COVID-19 data but also estimates risk.

The pandemic is also changing the rate at which data is being shared through other disciplines such as health geography. When data is publicized by countries, public web services become available that allow GIS users to consume data in creative formats. As a subsequent illustration, the World Health Organization (WHO) launched its COVID-19 dashboard that leverages GIS technology to display critical information across the globe in January of 2020, the same month as Johns Hopkins University. The dashboard depicts the entire globe. Users can click on any continent or country to gain more insight into COVID-19 details in that region.

Big problems also result in organic collaboration, consensus, and correction in the IT domain. Before February 18, 2020, the JHU and World Health Organization dashboards had several disparities such as the total number of COVID-19 cases. JHU used data from chest imaging and a symptom array in contrast to World Health Organization, which presented laboratory test results. However, a consensus was made on the optimal parameters for accurate case counts, resulting in both dashboards displaying the same number of cases (Kamel Boulos & Geraghty, 2020).

Data visualization is at the forefront of the COVID-19. As the latter examples indicate, how data is presented can lead to different interpretations. Incorrect interpretations undermine an individual's ability to assess therapeutic risk. In the future, world leaders and policymakers have a responsibility to ensure the accurate analysis and presentation of data. Transparency into the data, analysis, and visualizations is essential. Therefore, stronger international standards are necessary to safeguard the transition of data to information, knowledge, and wisdom.

IoTBDS and data visualization have played prominent roles in the struggle against COVID-19. However, beneath the vivid depictions of three-dimensional illustrations are two powerful components that enable their functionality—computer hardware and the data centers that power and connect this hardware.

COMPUTER HARDWARE

COVID-19 has amplified the role of computing hardware in our daily lives. The IoT, electronic cars, and outer space exploration are merely a few microcosms of the macro shift of human dependencies on computer hardware. IoT allows a home refrigerator to connect to the Internet. This connection opens the door for many other technological enhancements

Figure 7.1

COVID-19 Dashboard by the Center for Systems Science and Engineering at Johns Hopkins University

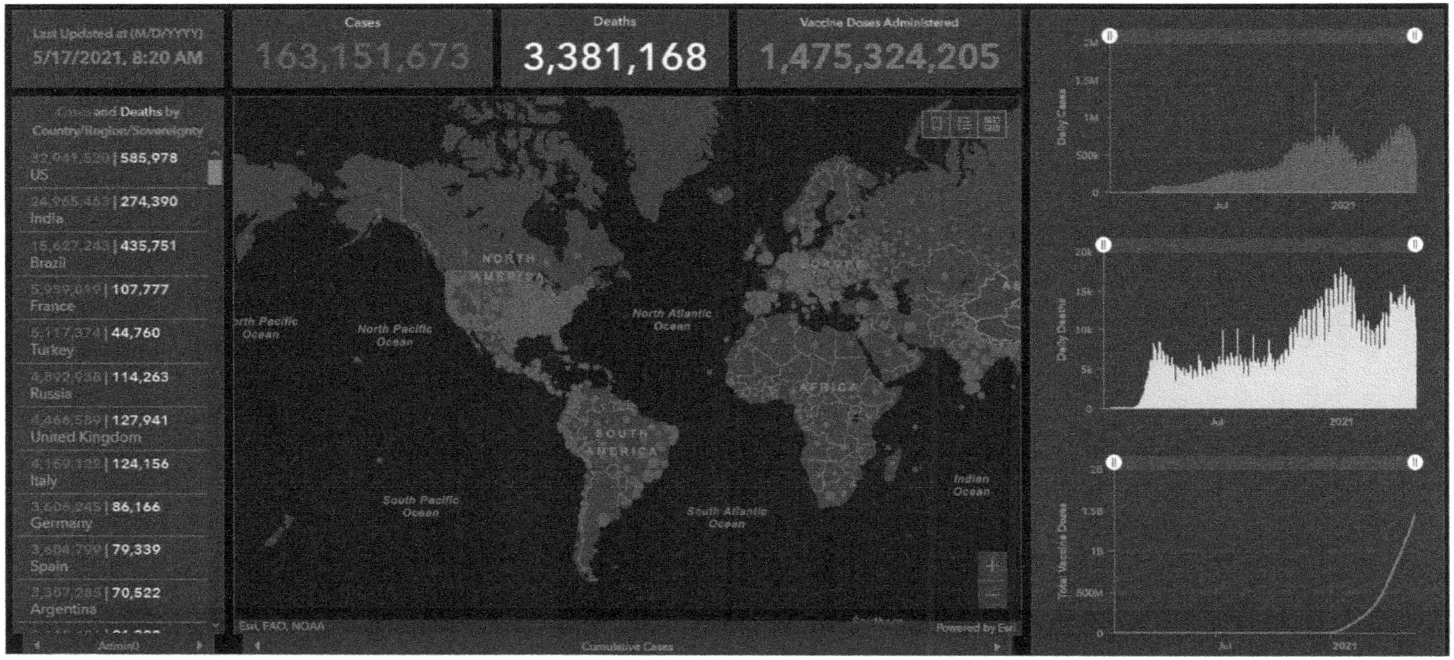

and communications. Today, artificial intelligence can predict inventory shortages and order new products when necessary. A future lifesaving capability is having medicine available as a result of rapid changes in demand that manufacturers can sense and respond to from refrigerator data. Similarly, as humanity depletes the resources of earth, space exploration holds valuable replacements. At the heart of space travel and exploration are computing control boards, which orchestrate everything from robotic movement to device communication. Despite our increasing reliance on computer hardware, recent supply chain problems emphasize the frailty of human dependency on hardware.

The world's primary suppliers of semiconductors have struggled immensely to keep up with demand during the COVID-19 pandemic. Accounting for exports and imports, semiconductors are the most traded product on earth after oil and vehicles. At the time of this writing, most electronic devices contain microcontrollers, which are in particularly short supply. Consumers are reporting half a year wait times or more for these parts (Jeong & Strumpf, 2021). Certain types of semiconductors have 1-year lead times (Vakil & Linton, 2021). The resulting bottlenecks in supply chains have baffled consumers.

The agility of supply chains continues to improve; however, this also has negative implications. In the auto industry, manufacturers quickly reduced their orders to many parts including semiconductors when vehicle sales dropped amidst the COVID-19 pandemic. When consumer demand returned, automakers were caught flat footed by semiconductor shortages. A series of unfortunate events in the supply chain further exacerbated the problem. Fires at several Japanese plants reduced production. U.S. and China trade relations also had rippling effects. In certain cases, companies that had predicted sales growth and/or were more agile, placed semiconductor orders prior to automakers (Jeong & Strumpf, 2021; Vakil & Linton, 2021).

At least one significant lesson are the weaknesses associated with human reliance on computing hardware. COVID-19 accentuates the critical dependencies on semiconductors. However, there are much greater implications for the future. As many computer scientists predict, Moore's Law will end. Moore observed that the number of transistors on a computer chip was doubling about every 18–24 months. This will require alternatives to silicon-based computing.

DATA CENTERS

Perhaps a lesser discussed yet certainly no less critical resource during pandemics are data centers (DCs). Data centers provide the facilities necessary to sustain large pools of interconnected computer hardware. DCs saw significant increases in their importance and utility during the COVID-19 pandemic. From their mission critical role of supporting intensive care units to an increased function of empowering social distancing by meeting the demands of virtualized meetings, events, and even sporting competitions, data centers are powering the virtual digitized realm of daily life during the pandemic (Westmattelmann et al., 2021; Wrycza & Maślankowski, 2020).

The pandemic resulted in a significant shift toward individuals becoming more reliant upon their home internet service provider. As employees traded their work office for home office, many saw significant changes in the speed at which they could complete their occupational responsibilities. Employees shifted from face-to-face office environments to virtual face-to-face video conferencing at home. Although web-conferencing systems had been prominent prior to the COVID-19 pandemic, their amount of use increased as companies moved employees to part-time or full-time remote working environments (Hacker et al., 2020). While many web-conferencing applications have similar graphical user interfaces regardless of physical location, the Internet connection speed on which they operate can change their effectiveness. Home computer networks are often much slower than enterprise-class communication networks and can be less reliable.

Due to data security, employees operating from home also faced clunkier technologies like virtual private networks, which further limits network bandwidth. Cloud applications can prevent the requirement of these cumbersome technologies; however, they have their own performance issues. Imagine relying on caffeine from a coffee shop inside a corporate office in contrast to a few miles away from a home office. Similarly, internal applications or client-side applications that use resources from a local data center have the capability to respond faster to user requests than remote cloud applications. Simply, cloud applications require additional network devices to relay traffic at greater distances. Data centers located in the same building and/or campus as employees naturally have greater bandwidth and less congestion due to competing network traffic across the Internet.

COVID-19 has resulted in significant shifts in where and how users connect to critical applications necessary in their daily lives. Prior to the pandemic, video streaming services had already forced considerable changes to DCs supporting public cloud services. However, working from home further elevated the need for corporate data centers to also evolve. As cloud applications grow, including the massive real time streaming of high-bandwidth content such as video, DCs must rapidly evolve. DCs suffer from several significant problems that are outpaced by other fundamental streaming technologies forced to progress during the COVID-19 pandemic such as microservices, application delivery networks, and content delivery networks. Nevertheless, attempting to make significant changes to data centers is like trying to turn a large ship around in a small harbor. Data centers change at a much slower pace than many other technologies (Darwesh et al., 2020).

While DC changes even amidst a pandemic are slow moving, their steady design and implementation set the stage for more agile and powerful big data systems. As one example, data center networks evolving over wireless signals has the potential to overcome certain physical and energy-based barriers. Simultaneous Transmission and Air Computation (STAC) in wireless data networks is an early proposed model. STAC advances software defined network architecture by integrating wireless transceivers into the communication network (Zhang et al., 2015). Wireless intra data center connections overcome several barriers to connecting new DCs quickly over wired connections. Free space optical communication is potential solution to requiring wired connections between new data centers (Darwesh et al., 2020).

As data center innovation accelerates, it will provide new opportunities for more significant compute power at lower costs and using less energy. Current cost centers that leverage DCs are cloud service providers. As data centers evolve, reliant high-level services like cloud computing are likely to be replaced by cheaper alternatives.

CLOUD COMPUTING

Unforgiving pandemics require scalable computing resources in a short amount of time. Cloud computing is now an established IT architecture that provides this capability. Cloud computing and/or an alternative IT architecture will provide more flexible and scalable resources for both small and large pandemics in the future. To illustrate a recent snapshot of this future potential, ventilator shortages presents a tremendous challenge with dire consequences during the COVID-19 pandemic. A recently proposed solution is for multiple patients to share one ventilator. However, this introduces many challenges. In an attempt to solve these problems, a team of clinicians and engineers at Duke University proposed a ventilator splitter and resistor system. The team leveraged cloud computing to design and test a model, scale the model, and generate a simulation of the model (Kaplan et al., 2021). Future pandemics will leverage cross-discipline teams with access to more computing power, solving larger problems faster. To better illustrate these evolving capabilities, consider how cloud computing currently operates.

Welsh and Benkhelifa (2020) define the cloud in context of two primary components, (1) cloud service providers (CSPs) and (2) service level agreements (SLAs). Cloud service providers host layers of computing hardware, networking, and software that allow end users to consume these resources without having to host them in their own data centers. DCs contain the physical infrastructure of cloud computing. This includes the computer networking hardware such as routers and switches. It contains the storage, such as massive storage area networks. Servers are a subsequent element. The second component defined, service level agreements, allow a package of computing and networking resources to be delivered to a consumer of the cloud at a cost. CSPs deliver optimal levels of computational service availability to their customers on the basis of service level agreements. For example, a service commitment of a CSP could be a minimum monthly uptime percentage of 99.99%. If the service level agreement is unmet due to associated hardware failures in the data center, customers receive a credit in some form (Welsh & Benkhelifa, 2020).

Beneficial to cloud computing is the ability to scale resources only when needed. Suppose that an event like the Olympics requires additional web services due to increased website traffic over a span of only a few months every 2 years. Cloud services prevent having additional data center resources such as power, servers, storage, and networking equipment to sit idle when demand is low. COVID-19 is a perfect scenario where cloud computing can benefit a large project with a finite timespan.

Recently, Michael Kaplan at the Duke University School of Medicine led a multidisciplinary team to create a lifesaving solution in a short amount of time—increasing ventilator capacity using massive parallel models of splitting. A critical challenge of the problem was the need to simulate hundreds of millions of clinical variations when splitting ventilators between COVID-19 patients with distinct respiratory physiologies. Cloud computing provided an avenue to solve this complex problem in a short timeline, resulting in the deployment of a capable IT architecture within 24 hours of the vision. In 72 hours, the implemented cloud computing environment had amassed 800,000 compute hours (Kaplan et al., 2021).

Cloud computing and/or its replacement will require data centers to connect more seamlessly and scale with greater elasticity. Similar to wireless antennas, this may require smaller data centers that are located closer to end users. Regardless of how these underlying IT infrastructures evolve, future pandemics will be met by larger research environments, greater computational power, and more accessible and collaborative cloud computing applications. A significant enabler of these advancements prior to and during the COVID-19 pandemic is the ever-increasing need for people to operate with flexibility and mobility.

MOBILITY

Mobile applications have emerged as powerful tools that can be developed swiftly to meet near immediate needs during the COVID-19 pandemic. Big data analytics using distributed and parallel computing are capable of delivering results quickly to end users. However, a distinct challenge once data is analyzed is ensuring the data is returned to the end user, such as the clinician, in a form that is easily understood, current, and accurate (Kaplan et al., 2021). Mobile applications have responded to several needs during the pandemic due to their effectiveness at reaching the greatest number of end users in the shortest amount of time.

Ingenuity of mobile developers has been on full display during the COVID-19 pandemic. Mobile applications developed to assist people include but are not limited to the following functionality:

- education and information;
- health assessment including self-monitoring capabilities;
- health monitoring leveraging technology like IoT to provide data to medical experts;
- hospital information;
- interactive reporting interfaces to share near real-time data on the pandemic;
- mental health support and data; and
- telehealth including specialties like teleophthalmology (Kondylakis et al., 2020).

Mobile applications give access to critical information in near real time for people, patients, healthcare professionals, the public sector, and private corporations. Applications exist that perform contact tracing, track symptoms, and help individuals receive access to proper care quickly through telehealth. Applications also provided notable resources for supporting mental health in a dark period of history (Kondylakis et al., 2020).

Mobile applications are reducing burdens on healthcare professionals, facilities, and supporting resources. Their future is bright as a primary front-end user interface that travels with people wherever they go. Despite their incredible utility to help during times of great duress, they are also a common mechanism used in some form by cybercriminals.

CYBERSECURITY

COVID-19 continues to underline the need for the public and private sectors to squash cyber-attacks that take advantage of vulnerable events and victims. From small businesses to large governments, cyber criminals have been very successful during the COVID-19 pandemic (Lallie et al., 2021; He et al., 2021; Tam et al., 2021). Following the first reported COVID-19 case in China, cybersecurity experts reported a significant pandemic-themed cyberattack within 30 days. A subsequent attack is reported to have occurred only 14 days later. Sadly, the timeline for cyberattacks shortened as cybercriminals began to take advantage of the associated weaknesses caused by the pandemic (Lallie et al., 2021). In a review of 39 key articles during the COVID-19 pandemic, Lallie et al., 2021 developed a timeline of cyberattacks throughout the world. Their research found 43 cyberattacks related to COVID-19, which are classified as:

- 37 were smishing or phishing;
- 28 were malware related;
- 15 associated with financial fraud;
- 6 included extortion;
- 6 involved pharming;
- 2 were denial of service attacks; and
- 2 were specific hacking events (Lallie et al., 2021, p. 10).

In the healthcare industry specifically, the pandemic highlights several critical areas of cyber awareness and necessary action starting with endpoint devices in computer networks. Any connected medical device or sensor, such as those present in patient-monitoring electronic hardware, are at risk of manipulation and/or takeover. IoT further accentuates the need for cybersecurity in healthcare. Ponder for a moment the effect of ransomware on life-saving intensive care units.

As merely one layer of the onion, endpoint security focuses on preventing and detecting intrusions on the outer network perimeters of a computer network. This layer of security is also capable of identifying when data is breached in healthcare facilities. Regardless of how secure a healthcare network perimeter is, where its local connections leave its internal network for the Internet, the internal network has its own vulnerabilities. Patient waiting rooms, for example, may have wireless access with vulnerable inroads into the hospital's network (He et al., 2021).

A subsequent and critical layer of cybersecurity is where people meet the associated technology. Human error and lack of security awareness remain the most significant vulnerabilities within the healthcare industry.

Phishing emails during the pandemic often targeted healthcare staff with access to critical patient data. The pandemic highlights the need for greater cyberawareness training, more significant funding for endpoint security, and larger cybersecurity teams in the healthcare industry to meet the increasing demands of information security (He et al., 2021).

FUTURE IMPLICATIONS OF IT AND PANDEMICS

Paramount to the future of computer and data sciences is a sufficient workforce. An increasingly discussed topic among higher education professionals is the decline of incoming student preparation in the core disciplines of science, technology, engineering, and math (STEM). While emphasis throughout the world is placed on science, technology, engineering, and math, it is insufficient. Concentrated and united efforts are necessary in the life cycle of education, from young to old.

The future of a trained workforce to help solve dire pandemics like COVID-19 is bright. IT continues to evolve due to the creativity and ingenuity of computer and data scientists. As we surpass Moore's Law, we will also advance beyond disruptive technologies like quantum computing. Although we cannot predict the new computational architecture that will replace classical computing, we see remnants of the needs it will need to meet. The pandemic highlights the demand for faster simulations for drug development, testing, approval, and distribution. Quantum artificial intelligence, quantum physics, semiconductor replacements, and/or similar disruptions have the potential to classify genomic data exponentially faster than classical computing architectures. In the interim, data centers and cloud computing are progressing to meet larger computational resource needs at scale in shorter periods of time. To facilitate this evolution, microservice architecture will need to be replaced with more agile, efficient, fault-tolerant, faster, and secure designs.

Artificial intelligence and machine learning are advancing through multiple sectors such as autonomous vehicles, which will help fund larger AI research efforts in healthcare. AI will be able to decipher emotions, symptoms, and countless other human attributes more accurately over time, leading to faster detection and prognosis of disease and mental health issues. Telehealth disruptions will increase healthcare accessibility, including connecting specialized physicians with patients less expensively and in shorter periods. Big data systems are advancing distributed and parallel computing, which allow deep learning algorithms faster access to larger amounts of data using thousands of interconnected servers. IoT, cloud computing, mobile applications, and WSNs provide future avenues to collect, analyze, and monitor near real time data streams from patients located throughout the universe. Data visualization will expand beyond modern dashboards using advancements from augmented and virtual reality to help medical professionals and patients make more informed decisions.

These are merely a few examples. While no technological disruption can counter the destruction of COVID-19, through the extraordinary efforts of humankind to advance innovative technologies, we can see moments of light protruding through the dark shadow cast by the ongoing pandemic.

REFERENCES

Chang, V., Muñoz, V. M., & Ramachandran, M. (2020). Emerging applications of internet of things, big data, security, and complexity: Special issue on collaboration opportunity for IoTBDS and COMPLEXIS. *Computing*, *102*(6), 1301–1304. https://doi.org/10.1007/s00607-020-00811-y

Darwesh, L., Arnon, S., & Kopeika, N. (2020). Characterization of free space optical data center channel. *Microwave and Optical Technology Letters*, *62*(9), 3087–3094. https://doi.org/10.1002/mop.32418

ElDahshan, K. A., AlHabshy, A. A., & Abutaleb, G. E. (2020). Data in the time of COVID-19: A general methodology to select and secure a NoSQL DBMS for medical data. *PeerJ Computer Science*. Coronavirus Research Database; ProQuest Central; SciTech Premium Collection. https://doi.org/10.7717/peerj-cs.297

Faculty Lauren Gardner. (n.d.). *Bio*. https://engineering.jhu.edu/case/faculty/lauren-gardner/

Jeong, E., & Strumpf, D. (2021, April). Why the chip shortage is so hard to overcome. https://www.wsj.com/articles/why-the-chip-shortage-is-so-hard-to-overcome-11618844905

Hacker, J., vom Brocke, J., Handali, J., Otto, M., & Schneider, J. (2020). Virtually in this together—How web-conferencing systems enabled a new virtual togetherness during the COVID-19 crisis. *European Journal of Information Systems*, *29*(5), 563–584. https://doi.org/10.1080/0960085X.2020.1814680

He, Y., Aliyu, A., Evans, M., & Luo, C. (2021). Health care cybersecurity challenges and solutions under the climate of COVID-19: Scoping review. *Journal of Medical Internet Research*, *23*(4), e21747. https://doi.org/10.2196/21747

Kamel Boulos, M. N., & Geraghty, E. M. (2020). Geographical tracking and mapping of coronavirus disease COVID-19/severe acute respiratory syndrome coronavirus 2 (SARS-CoV-2) epidemic and associated events around the world: How 21st century GIS technologies are supporting the global fight against outbreaks and epidemics. *International Journal of Health Geographics*, *19*(1), 1–12. https://doi.org/10.1186/s12942-020-00202-8

Kaplan, M., Kneifel, C., Orlikowski, V., Dorff, J., Newton, M., Howard, A., Shinn, D., Bishawi, M., Simbarashe, C., Balogh, P., & Randles, A. (2021). A cloud-based data collaborative to combat the COVID-19 pandemic and to solve major technology challenges. *Future Internet*, *13*(3), 37–47. https://doi.org/10.3390/fi13030061

Kondylakis, H., Katehakis, D. G., Kouroubali, A., Logothetidis, F., Triantafyllidis, A., Kalamaras, I., Votis, K., & Tzovaras, D. (2020). COVID-19 mobile apps: A systematic review of the literature. *Journal of Medical Internet Research*, *22*(12), e23170. https://doi.org/10.2196/23170

Lallie, H. S., Shepherd, L. A., Nurse, J. R. C., Erola, A., Epiphaniou, G., Maple, C., & Bellekens, X. (2021). Cyber security in the age of COVID-19: A timeline and analysis of cyber-crime and cyber-attacks during the pandemic. *Computers & Security*, *105*, 102248. https://doi.org/10.1016/j.cose.2021.102248

Li, W., Chai, Y., Khan, F., Jan, S. R. U., Verma, S., Menon, V. G., Kavita, & Li, X. (2021). A comprehensive survey on machine learning-based big data analytics for IoT-enabled smart healthcare system. *Mobile Networks and Applications*, *26*(1), 234–252. https://doi.org/10.1007/s11036-020-01700-6

Tam, T., Rao, A., & Hall, J. (2021). The invisible COVID-19 small business risks: Dealing with the cyber-security aftermath. *Digital Government: Research and Practice*, *2*(2). https://doi.org/10.1145/3436807

Vakil, B., & Linton, T. (2021, February). Why we're in the midst of a global semiconductor shortage. *Harvard Business Review*. https://hbr.org/2021/02/why-were-in-the-midst-of-a-global-semiconductor-shortage#

Welsh, T., & Benkhelifa, E. (2020). On resilience in cloud computing: A survey of techniques across the cloud domain. *ACM Computing Surveys*, *53*(3). https://doi.org/10.1145/3388922

Westmattelmann, D., Grotenhermen, J.-G., Sprenger, M., & Schewe, G. (2021). The show must go on—Virtualisation of sport events during the COVID-19 pandemic. *European Journal of Information Systems*, *30*(2), 119–136. https://doi.org/10.1080/0960085X.2020.1850186

Wrycza, S., & Maślankowski, J. (2020). Social media users' opinions on remote work during the COVID-19 pandemic. *Information Systems Management*, *37*(4), 288–297. https://doi.org/10.1080/10580530.2020.1820631

Zhang, S., Wu, X., & Ozgur, A. (2015). STAC: Simultaneous transmitting and air computing in wireless data center networks. *2015 IEEE/CIC International Conference on Communications in China*, 1–7. https://doi.org/10.1109/ICCChina.2015.7448704

CHAPTER 8

NETWORKING POSTPANDEMIC JUST GOT EASIER *AND* HARDER

Clay Morgan

INTRODUCTION

Business networking is vital to your success. It does not matter if you are an introvert or extrovert. From connections and clients to tips and tools, networking provides opportunities and wisdom that keep countless businesses and business leaders on track. But how do you network when *everyone* is in forced isolation? That is the question we had to answer in March of 2020.

Our organization, BNI, had over 250,000 members in over 70 countries at that time. That is over one quarter of a million business professionals who became members of our organization to network and pass business referrals. They all met locally to network once a week.

For our 35 year existence as a company, we always met in the same format to network. We met in person. We shook hands and shared hugs. We exchanged connections and ideas across the table while we shared coffee or a meal. Then, we came face to face with a global health pandemic.

NETWORKING ONLINE—A NECESSARY SHIFT

Like so many hurdles forced in all our paths by the pandemic, we found solutions. In this case, our solution started with setting up *lots* of zoom

Back to a New Normal: In Search of Stability in an Era of Pandemic Disruption—Insight From Practitioners and Academics, pp. 111–117

licenses and optimizing our resources so our weekly networking meetings would work smoothly in an online setting. Once we had the infrastructure set, we moved all our networking operations from in-person to online. This was an imperative move for our members' businesses and for the local economies where they live.

Networking has a significant impact on our economy. Knowing that our members generated over $16.5 billion worth of business for each other in 2019 (prior to the pandemic), we felt an intense responsibility to keep the wheels of business networking on the tracks. During a time when so many things were uncertain and many businesses were faltering, we had to provide a solution to continue generating results for our members and their businesses.

The ripple effect within companies and communities would be large either way. The question was, will this necessary shift to networking online work, especially given the economic constraints from the pandemic which were beyond our control?

Fast forward through 2020 (something you may wish you could do entirely) and we found our answer to the question of whether shifting all our networking online would work. Our clients generated $17.5 billion in revenue through referrals for one another by networking in 2020. That is $1 billion more revenue than the year before!

Keep in mind we were not just networking online for the convenience of avoiding traffic or trading in professional attire for more casual clothes and slippers. For large parts of the year, everyone was in forced quarantine or had limited opportunity for typical in person connections with clients, family, and friends. In our company's 35 years of history prior to the pandemic, we have always met to network in person and pass business referrals. Our first year networking online, members set a record for revenue generated. This makes a strong case that networking online can be effective.

NETWORKING—A NEW NORMAL?

This begs the question, "Now that isolation is not required, how do we establish the "new normal for networking?" Are we better off doing all networking remotely or are we better off knowing we made the most of an unforgettable challenge but make the shift back to traditional in-person networking?

There will be some professionals who will lean heavily on the side of online networking and proclaim it as the way of the future. Other professionals will lean on the side of a return to all in-person networking going forward because they believe networking online was simply the best we could do at the time. Now that we are able to safely network in—person, that is what we should do because online is a good back-up option, but it should be just that—a backup option.

With my experience operating in-person networking and the online networking, I can comfortably tell you that the pandemic has changed networking forever. It showed us how networking can be done more *easily* than ever before. Like many changes though, this increased capability will make some aspects of networking *harder* than they were prior to the pandemic.

ON SUCCESSFUL NETWORKING

Here are the four things business leaders need to know to network successfully—in an increasing order of importance—going forward:

#4: Networking Online Is Here to Stay

Networking online allows you to reach more people, more often. The pandemic has proven that we can connect and network effectively online and avoid some of the traditional constraints of in-person networking events. For example, when you network online through a meeting being held on Zoom or Go to Meeting, you do not have to drive or fly to a specific location. This saves time and money, especially if you are the one paying for a venue. If you are hosting a networking meeting, the size of the venue also impacts your maximum number of attendees. When networking online, those constraints and limitations all but disappear. From the standpoint of cost opportunity and time invested in travel, online networking provides significant benefits which organizations and individuals alike will keep for the long term.

You might be thinking that online meeting platforms like Zoom and Go to Meeting were available prior to the pandemic, and networking events were not wildly popular then. You are correct. However, the difference is mass adoption. In any industry, the success of an innovation relies on the company's ability to influence the market to try the new offering rather than simply selecting the product they are used to. When it comes to mass adoption of online networking using platforms like the ones mentioned above, the challenge prior to the pandemic was a lack urgency.

In-person networking was the standard and it worked. There were several meetings held online with them, but few with the intent of interactive networking the way you typically would at an event in a hotel ballroom or a mixer in the back room of a local restaurant. The other reason there was not a mass adoption of online networking before is that it was one more thing to adopt! You had to download and learn a new software program, understand how to use your webcam, and … why would you do that when you could just go to an event?

The pandemic created a tipping point that has brought online networking here to stay because there were no in-person networking events to go to. As a professional, you had to learn to adopt the tools to network successfully, or not network. Going forward, the capabilities of these platforms will continue to expand and improve. This will allow younger generations entering the workforce to connect with older generations more readily in the workforce and help both bridge the communication gap while leveraging these tools and innovations.

#3: In-Person Networking Will Become a Richer, More Valuable Experience

While I am excited that online networking is here to stay, please understand that is I do not believe in-person networking is going away. Quite the opposite. I believe in person networking will be more valued than ever. Think about how many times during the pandemic you heard or said, "This whole situation really puts things in perspective and makes you feel grateful for what you have." I do not know the exact number, but I'm guessing it was approximately *a lot* of times!

You said it because it was true. It was true about health, family, friends, and work. It was true about connecting with other people! In the context of our conversation here about networking, that means we were grateful for the opportunity to continue connecting with and networking with others through these online platforms during the pandemic. However grateful we were though, there was one thing that was undeniable. You cannot shake somebody's hand online. You cannot give a beloved colleague a hug or share a high five with a fellow business owner you're trading business referrals with when you're on a screen.

There is a certain energy, a certain magic, a certain experience we all have when we share the same physical space. It is simply undeniable. When you are in a room networking with 30, 50 75, or 100 people, it has a different energy in-person than it does online. In the same way watching your favorite football team play on TV while sitting in your favorite chair is different than watching them from great seats halfway up the lower bowl on the 50 yard, so it is with networking.

There is less traffic, more convenience, and easier access to the bathroom, but it is an undeniably different experience. That is why so many folks enjoy watching games from home but relish those times when they get to go to the stadium and cheer their team on in-person. A big part of why attending games or networking events in-person just has the little something extra is because of the connection to the other people in the room or in the stadium. Again, online events are very effective, and it does create a shared experience, but we are still experiencing it differently than when we're in the same room.

#2: Pick the Combination of Networking Events That Will Be Most Beneficial for You

One of the traps that will emerge in networking because of the pandemic is that some professionals will attend one type of networking event —only online or only in person. Avoid the trap! People will have their own preference when it comes to networking formats but recognize that there is not one "best format".

Thanks to the pandemic we now have the luxury to have more dynamic in-person meetings rather than taking that format for granted. We can truly embrace the experience of connecting with other people in the same room rather than the same screen. We can also recapture time and create different networking experiences online. Do both with intentionality!

One comment about networking I heard from a number of folks during the pandemic was "Thank goodness for online networking. Now I'll never have to go back to mastering the art of how to break into a group conversation or making awkward small talk during mixers." Some of these folks may be introverts who do not prefer crowded events or highly task-oriented individuals who do not feel small talk is a good use of their time.

In any case, their desires for simplified networking are well and good. Unfortunately for them though, they are only desires. Wishful thinking. That is because in any format, networking is still about talking with people to create a personal connection and develop a relationship over time. The same dance takes place when networking online. The steps just look and feel a little different. Also, when you are networking online, you probably will not need to ask for directions or run into a long line if you need to go to the bar or the bathroom.

Your approach to networking varies from others you know based on your industry, your role in your company, and even your behavioral style. While these variables may change the lens through which you "see" networking and how to network, it imperative that you are intentional about picking the right balance of in-person networking opportunities and online networking opportunities. Simply put, there are people who you would not meet otherwise or be able to connect with if you only stick to one format.

#1: Be Present Where You Are

In our electronic age, the state of constant distraction is a societal norm. From social media apps pushing notifications to grab our attention to constantly checking emails, text messages, slack notifications, and more... there are so many distractions literally at our fingertips every waking hour.

Whether it is in a professional setting or a personal setting, we all wrestle with being present thanks to constant availability and access. Thanks to the pandemic, we saw the state of constant distraction to creep further into networking.

When you attend a networking meeting with dozens of other professionals in the banquet hall at a local restaurant, you don't expect one of the people you are having a conversation within a small group of 3 people to pull out their phone and begin replying to email or chat messages.

It may happen rarely, especially if someone is expecting a call from a loved one or an emergency at the office, but you certainly don't expect it. When you are having a conversation at a networking event, everyone is there for the same reason and typically honors the others time. They stay present at the event.

As networking pressed online in mass due to the pandemic, networking from home or your office meant sitting in front of a computer screen. Perhaps two or three computer screens. This forces you to be very intentional about ignoring the whirlwind all around you, being readily available and even notifying you right there on your screen about other tasks. This is one of the greatest challenges of online networking. It is that you are online.

Certainly, you can turn everything else on your device off, but it requires discipline. That is because you are not transitioning to a new setting. Your brain is not resetting and adapting to a new environment.

When you go to a traditional in-person networking event, you may take calls on your way to the meeting, but you spend time traveling to the event. Subconsciously, your brain knows you are in transit to do something else. Once you arrive, you put the phone, tablet, or laptop away so you can network. Even if your phone buzzes during the meeting, it is in your purse or pocket. You know to check it after the meeting.

You also know you are sharing the same meeting space with other professionals who will see you check your phone in front of them, signaling that there is something more important than being there. The social expectations of the situation allow or force you to be present.

When networking online, your brain does not get that time or physical space in the car to transition. You are still in front of the same screen where you reply to customer messages, communicate with your team, check your social media, and keep all your digital files. Your ability to be present for an online networking meeting is directly proportional to your discipline and will power to completely ignore all those windows which are right in front of you, behind the faces you are networking with on the screen. In either format being present is the most important thing. The format of the meeting is secondary.

NETWORKING—OPPORTUNITIES AND BENEFITS

Both online networking and in-person networking have incredible benefits. Both work. It has never been *easier* to network than today and going forward. Between tried and true in person networking opportunities and now a mass adoption of online networking tools, you truly have more opportunities to cultivate meaningful connections efficiently.

What makes networking work is that it is an opportunity to create connection. Connection is one of your most essential needs you have as a human being. When you connect with other human beings, it provides you the opportunity to grow. It enables you to grow by tapping into the knowledge and resources of others who are different from you. It enables you to share your knowledge and resources with others. That combination of giving and receiving is life giving.

However, networking only works when you work it. If professionals become too distracted to really work a room—online or in-person, it will not create connection. We had enough distractions in our life before the pandemic creating a disconnection. We now have an opportunity to make sure technology enhances real life interaction. That will make networking easier. The danger is not letting technology overtake it. That will make it *harder*.

CHAPTER 9

PANDERING TO PANDEMICS

Framing Choices for Success—Insights for CEOs

Lathan Craig Austin

INTRODUCTION

This chapter explores how cognitive structures or schema (how we make sense of things around us) are used in organizations to perceive, interpret, and act on environmental cues that managers must examine as part of maintaining the firm's performance metrics, especially during times of a pandemic.

Normally, businesses get surprised with the disruptive innovations (the first iPhone) or disruptive technologies (the calculator over the slide rule; the digital camera over using film), but the pandemic has created an even more fundamental challenge: a disruptive environment that many organizations are finding it difficult to compete in. Some firms have been nimble or agile enough to respond strategically, such as ConAgra, which has marketed and modernized some of its recipes and packaging across the Marie Callender's and Healthy Choice brands, betting that consumers will continue cooking and lunching at home for the near future.

Back to a New Normal: In Search of Stability in an Era of Pandemic Disruption—Insight From Practitioners and Academics, pp. 119–131

THE NEW NORMAL

Kraft-Heinz has invested its monies into expanding its higher demand products such as Kraft Mac & Cheese cups and Oscar Mayer cold cuts while others such as PepsiCo has reduced 20% of its product offerings so as to focus on just the faster moving items. Since World War II the strategy of adding an ever-increasing number of product choices to appeal to every possible consumer segment was the enduring corporate mantra, evidenced in how Lays Potato Chips increased its available selections from its first four items 45 years ago to at least 60 products as of 2020. Campbell Soup has currently about 400 different soups it markets (Gasparro & Terlep, 2020). The philosophy traditionally employed has increasingly been a meal for any and every customer.

The panic buying that cleaned out store shelves in March of 2020 gave most retail executives some pause in deciding what to produce and for how long. Americans had become addicted to having endless varieties, whether it be chips or soups, which has simply stressed factories and overwhelmed the capacity of stores. Pleasing every customer became very difficult in the pandemic because consumer demand was shifting away from past buying levels and away from particular brands. Simultaneously, logistics providers have struggled with tepid recoveries of supply items while there has been ongoing demand destruction. BestBuy, though riding a tremendous wave of homebound consumers buying televisions and other electronic equipment, is still banking that the prepandemic trend will continue to shift toward online purchasing, virtual technology services, and smaller stores.

While it is clear that consumer habits are in transition, the pandemic has also lasted long enough to make some of those habits more predictable to anticipate. Uber and DoorDash continue to pick up restaurant orders and various grocery stores deliver online orders to individual homes, which is not expected to change much, given consumers are both fearful and have too much money they cannot spend yet. Amazon, which stumbled at the beginning of the epidemic due to its strategy of maintaining very tight inventories, may yet obtain 25% of all e-commerce sales from a level of just 4% last year if its numbers continue to improve, thanks to robust consumer habits formed during the various lockdowns. Sales at Home Depot too, are quite strong versus those at Macy's, whose apparel sales fell 30% (Nassauer, 2021).

Many remote-working individuals have purchased devices or computer equipment that will enable them to work from their homes indefinitely so firms can have some confidence that some of the new changes in demand are here to stay. It is estimated that as much as 25% of all Americans will be home at least for a few days a week throughout 2021, such as

Alphabet's Google, compared to the previous 4% before the pandemic began. Indeed, many homes have undergone significant changes during the pandemic that they now serve simultaneously as offices, schools, and even small villages. This transformation has serious implications for how and in what direction our societies and economies may yet shift in the next few years. Cherished human habits of buying things as we find them and working in an office have broken apart such that a new way of operating for many has been initiated. Office towers will largely remain vacant or repurposed, as there is an unmistakable new business imprint or model being transposed onto the economy.

HOW ORGANIZATIONS THINK

How are some organizations able to navigate an environment as chaotic and unplanned as the one that is now mired in this pandemic? Drawing on an evolutionary process, corporate strategies are often formulated on how the "knowledge structure" or schema of an organization, its mental template, perceives its external environment, which is then recorded, interpreted in light of prior experiences, inferences are drawn, and a strategic response is crafted. These knowledge structures can be conceived as script tracks that consist of the objects, images, memories, et cetera, that are utilized as tools to help resolve the firm's problems that come up. For General Mills, this means that its effort to improve the quality of its Cheerios by adding more protein and reducing the sugar in its Yoplait yogurt is consistent with its traditional perception of its environment. The corporation, a big food maker, believes its customers will be home more and seeking to better manage the financial strains of the pandemic so it is in an enviable position to attract millions of new consumers to its products.

The concept of a "thinking" organization is more than simply a metaphor as it represents an understanding of an organization as a fountain of knowledge that is fed by its strategic decisions and the learning of the firm. Such thinking is largely done and finds its ablest expression in the actions of the firm's corporate elites. For organizations, deciphering the managerial cognition perspective is about understanding how managers scan their environment, process, and disseminate data based on prior experiences, derive insights into potential threats and opportunities, even during pandemics, and problem-solve current and future issues. For example, gyms have greatly suffered with this pandemic due to social distancing and may enjoy a much smaller footprint in the future. Peloton bikes and Nautilus, however, have recognized an opportunity and are expanding due to their being used by those who cannot access a gym now. These consumers are relishing these more creative, even superior, digitally connected ways to stay fit while at home, including attending virtual classes.

A competitive environment in the midst of a pandemic is simultaneously ambiguous, ever shifting, and extraordinarily complex for executives to decipher or make sense. As a result, organizations construct "frames" in order to interpret events both in order to make speedy decisions and to respond nimbly to changes in consumer demand (Fiss & Zajac, 2006). What are the frames corporate elites have adopted or will need to adopt from their learning in this environment?

Amazon has more employees than its competitors, but they require little training given the algorithms and automation it constructs to manage and direct its people. For example, a cloud-connected scanning gun observes the speed at which a warehouse worker picks up items, how many breaks he or she takes, and how accurate the worker is in choosing the right items and placing them where they need to be. Sellers too, are managed largely by automation software and are delisted without warning. Amazon uses this AI and its cloud-computing infrastructure to frame how it sees it must manage its workers and sellers in order to stay competitive while still creating a meaningful buying experience for its consumers (Mims, 2021).

Organizations actually undergo cognitive reframing at the same time as they undertake strategy shifts and amend internal processes (Sandberg & Tsoukas, 2015). Nestlé SA is reducing its Lean Cuisine varieties due to production difficulties, IGA is slicing its forty varieties of toilet paper it carries to just four, partly due to reliability problems with suppliers, while Georgia-Pacific devotes its production to larger sheet rolls that allow it to be more efficient and keep corporate clients happier as it better keeps the toilet paper in stock.

Many restaurants such as MacDonald's and Darden's have pared down their menus, keeping a number of offerings off, which has reduced prep work and costs, while noticeably increasing their speed of service. The image they hold of themselves and the brand they project is still making meals for any conceivable participating customer. Products have always imbued both a social and psychological facet that was strongly linked to its physical nature as well. The image consumers have about their brands, expressed in those feelings, beliefs, ideas, and attitudes they direct to these brands, are crucial to understanding what they choose to purchase. Organizations understand this psychology and construct strategies that allow them to better profit from the perception of their identities and image.

Such activities are often described as "sensemaking" and they are tied to how firms construct their marketplace identity and image. Stories of the firm's founding, myths of its dynamic history, etc. illustrate how these cognitive schemas are assembled. Members of an organization imbue this cognitive content or culture as it is sometimes described into the fabric of the firm. Weick (1995) posits that corporate decision-making is essentially sensemaking at work.

CONSTRUCTING NEW STRATEGIES OF SURVIVAL

Perception is after all a social experience. The content of the perceptual screens is defined and influenced by the world and the people around us. It is almost always collaborative. Managers both manufacture and maintain meaning within a firm. It can be argued that knowledge structures are most susceptible to change with pressures from the environment, sociopolitical processes at work, and a change in the beliefs, values, or assumptions of the management team. This is evident with Amazon, which struggles with its unions, who want to reduce Amazon's automation effects on the work of its employees, seen in its desire to implement automated drone deliveries. Its sellers sometimes find Amazon is also their competitor, but they are unable to walk away.

That these knowledge structures shift is never truer for an organization than when a management team is struggling with trying to understand its environment and actually make sense of it. How a manager chooses strategy and formulates goals and analysis depends on how he perceives his world and the cognitive structure around him. Indeed, organizations are interpretive by nature (Daft & Weick, 1984). They are also mental entities that engage in thinking where firms represent a sort of sociocognitive connectedness. For example, in order to reduce costs and increase profits, both Facebook and Lyft try to identify workers, who may work remotely from states where they do not have a legal presence. This allows them to reduce their salaries, which the pandemic helped reveal this necessity.

The framing of data or information that arrives at the firm elevates its decision-making. First, there is theory that argues that each industry both defines what is acceptable and also creates rules for the game under foot for its firms. This suggests these rules or "industry recipes" or cognitive bookmarks are specific enough that all firms choose to follow them. For example, the Scottish-knitwear makers follow the common rules of other knitwear makers in their country. Their supply chain partners build too, relationships based around these very same industry-type recipes of how to do things, such they tend to all work together.

This suggests that such cognition or "beliefs" about perceived relationships between information and concepts are what enable managers to make decisions. There were actual constraints to the reach of human rationality such that many environmental cues coming into the firm are unable to be understood or interpreted as needed by managers. The corporate belief system that frames incoming data includes the firm's identity, its competitors, its vendors, and its customers that provide a river of market cues to decipher and helps optimize decision-making. Per upper echelon views, it is the senior managers who scrutinize the information and craft an interpretation that precedes organizational action. J.M. Smucker has opportunistically reengaged its idled machines and reorganized its other equipment so as to produce its Folgers and Dunkin' coffee in quantities and varieties that it hopes will be popular with remote workers.

Business competition intertwines the material transactions occurring between the firm and the supply chain with the cognitive insights into competitor strategies and tactics to form a mental model for organizational elites of what it takes to succeed. Put differently, the organization remembers its past through its employees, the culture, structures, and processes of the firm where it can employ this memory in making strategic decisions. Firms also differ in their style of acquiring and utilizing data, which helps explain different outcomes and market positions. Clorox is counting on workers returning to their offices so it thinks sales will expand as workers will want to clean and disinfect their public workspaces.

Group cognitive structures often rise out of group-member interactions and debates where causal maps are thus created and agreed upon. Such group processes and interactions change what individuals may think and the resulting total is not necessarily the sum of the parts since the parts too, are in the midst of moving or changing. What emerges is a cognitive ability among firms in an industry that raises the quality of decision-making since the cognitive complexity present, especially in ambiguous environments, may necessitate greater coverage, diversity, or depth of group perspectives and experiences. Such diverse viewpoints within groups augment their ability in rather fundamental ways that improves decisions. Amy's Kitchen, a diverse management group, sees the pandemic an opening to construct a factory in San Jose, CA, and another on the east coast by next year so as to produce more of its organic soups and frozen meals that have done so well in sales during the pandemic.

MANAGEMENT AT WORK

Management teams both construct and maintain meaning within a firm. It can be argued it is one of the key tasks for a chief executive officer (CEO) to scan, interpret, and build a narrative around which the firm can draw or project identity both outward and inward. It is not just mere rhetoric to the industry or to supply chain stakeholders. This is best captured by Berger and Luckmann (1967) much earlier when they argued that what constitutes reality are the previous external projections of ideas that later became objectified behavior. This suggests that corporate managers draw ideas from their environment no matter how new they may seem to be. Outback Steakhouse has removed approximately 40% of its menu, as it perceives the environment as saying customers may not care and could even cut some items for good even after the pandemic.

Managers even choose language so that their environmental interpretations can influence the organizational perceptions of others. Some enforce their schemas through direct influence or decree such that firm schemas are changed as well. One of the most recognizable aspects of constructing meaning is the use of image as both an internal and external manifestation of how the firm wants to be understood by both themselves and others. Many agree that image is essentially a communicated concept. Similarly, strategies represent how the management team will interpret important issues that arise out of the environment. German corporations demonstrate how their adoption of shareholder value orientations was calculated as a means of using sensemaking to adapt to shareholder concerns.

Culture is often thought of as shared systems of meaning, which suggests that culture is also a cognition structure. Within a firm's culture are all the stories, myths, ways of doing things, and beliefs about themselves and others that represent cognition at the organizational level. Cultures are nurtured by management, but also amended as needed to reflect company goals and aspirations. Clearly, individuals vary in terms of the degree to which they embrace a firm's culture. Cultures also prescribe and socialize acceptable behavior and outlooks from employees. Though nonunionized, UPS is known for how it both draws from and amends its culture in order to pursue a value discipline of efficiency in its marketplace.

BEING NIMBLER AND MORE PRODUCTIVE

Whether they be cognition, knowledge structures, schema, causal maps, or cognitive scripts, they are all linked to firm performance. Firms are more than the carefully planned symbols constructed by them, the stock price that measures them, or the sum of their individual parts, which constitutes their identity, as viewed by others. Framing strategic changes entails the proposing of a new rendering of reality that draws in important stakeholders, including employees, to support the proposed change in course (Hänggli, 2020). Penske Logistics draws on its various stakeholders to better frame its view that both its suppliers and its shippers want to increase and vary their storage capacity closer to their customers instead of using massive warehouses in remote areas of the country.

A key task for any organization is how it manages corporate symbols and the interpretation of events on behalf of different, interested groups. Similarly, firm competition presents such a fundamental, even seismic, threat to the continued well-being of the firm. How managers perceive their rivals, resolve disruptions or discontinuities in the marketplace, and interpret environmental cues that necessitate action determines how well the firm performs. What is also interesting in understanding how causal maps of corporate managers work is that these maps change often, given their respond to changes in the competitive environment, which changes the frames of reference of these managers. The management group becomes increasingly proficient, thus improving performance. There is no better represented than with industrial real-estate giant, Prologis Inc., where its managers' maps change as they note businesses are acquiring new space so as to modernize their distribution operations, including being nearer to large urban areas.

Much of the previous thought on managerial cognition has suggested that organizations needed to have rich, even complex knowledge structures in order to be nimble enough to deal with an intensely changing market environment. Managers in these firms employ strategic schemas, the knowledge structures that the senior management group employs, to filter out irrelevant or extraneous information, diagnose problems in a too-ambiguous environment, and then adopt competitive behaviors that were geared toward improving performance. Consumer-products giant, Reckitt Benckiser, constructs good plans and forecasts, 6 months in advance, because decisions involving global production, recruiting, and other issues demand significant lead time. For example, its Lysol brand has done well during the pandemic, but its Durex condoms requires the bars and restaurants to reopen.

What few studies there are do not associate this cognition with firm performance though there are many, many firms in these highly competitive industries where the varying capabilities they possess or acquire are essential for their survival. They employ various sets of innovative and diverse actions that make possible new competitive posturing. What thinking made this possible? How did so many become so strategically flexible toward their market environment? Strategic schemas do matter for firm performance. They influence firm performance by putting forth meaningful strategic actions. Managers who fail to notice environmental shifts are less likely to act by changing the organization's strategic actions and respond timely. This showed how the relationship between strategic schemas, strategic flexibility, and performance demonstrate that strategic actions do mediate between strategic schemas and performance.

THE PRICE OF FAILURE

Knowledge structures are amendable. Their content often depends on social interaction patterns and communication within a firm or a major management shakeup that elicits new outlooks. Much of the research also suggests that change occurs as a result of discontinuities in the external environment (Christensen & Raynor, 2003). These could be technological breakthroughs that fundamentally shift how an industry is organized and does business, resource constraints that shift causal maps, or they could also be political in nature where changes in regulations transform an industry radically. Israel, which leads the world in vaccinating its citizens, has seen its domestic hotel bookings increase significantly, which portends well for manufacturers, such as those as Lysol, as the new wellness habits will continue when the pent-up demand is unleashed.

The price of not responding to such discontinuities can be quite high in terms of the survival of the firm. Changes in the information environments of CEOs resulted in transformations of their collective frames of reference or cognitive structures. Given how complex and difficult to decipher information coming into a firm can be for managers, this suggests a better knowledge structure for a firm would be one that encourages organizational action that can in turn facilitate corporate learning. In many ways, it is the action that the firm initiates that defines it and allows it to learn and to reinvent itself as needed to survive in its highly competitive environment. Qurate Retail that owns HSN and QVC have delayed workplace return dates until at least the summer, as it has been difficult for managers to interpret accurately the market in order to keep employees informed. Fidelity Investments also struggles with how to strategize in this market but keeps its employees in the dark as to when they can return.

This suggests also that complex strategic schemas allow greater selections of possible strategy solutions, which allow better decision-making and increased recognition of opportunities that makes the firm increasingly more adaptable. It is found that the greater the knowledge structures the greater the innovation and invention that firms could muster, which led to increased capacity to implement new ideas. The very concept of complexity suggests there are various degrees of depth for schemas and therefore such schemas are amenable. Alphabet's Google continues to delay the return of its workers until the fall, which illustrates how even some of the biggest corporations have trouble being adaptable enough to this environment.

Another aspect of strategic schemas that deserves some consideration is the extent that it is "focused" schema or centered on a handful of concepts, important to the firm. Such schemas tend to be associated with older, more stable, hierarchical firms, who have debated, elaborated, and cherished these beliefs over much time. What core set of knowledge structures that do evolve lend themselves to a narrow set of strategic decisions and actions. Such schemas resist amending. While there is some debate that firms with simpler or fewer knowledge structures or routines might enable them to respond and acquire new eventlike knowledge by experimenting in fast-moving industries, others have concluded that complex schemas with their varied store of images can better employ sensemaking that makes them more adaptive. Movie theatre chains and the studios, such as Universal and Disney, have more focused schema, which shows in their limited planning for reopening and their continued interest primarily in video streaming.

Cognitive structures are prisms from which management groups surveil their environments. This suggests also that these management groups have perceptual limits that impede digestion of environmental cues that must be recognized and translated into meaning in order for the organization to obtain and act on market intelligence. Perhaps, this is best illustrates by reexamining cognitive communities of the Scottish knitwear producers, who shared beliefs or constructed a mental model about how they defined themselves, who their competitors were, and who were their customers that framed how they looked at the competitive environment in which they were engaged.

LEARNING TO FRAME CHANGE

Frames are simply schemata of interpretation that condense the world into digestible bits that allow meaning to be constructed by elites for various audiences. Strategic plans that effectively embody the firm's view of its environment are essentially cognitive structures at work. What emerges as strategy or decision-making is often unintended given the blending that comes forth from both environment and corporate bureaucracy impacting one another in sometimes unpredictable, diverse ways. In many ways, organizations that adapt to competitive threats or environmental challenges suggests that there is indeed cognition underway within and across firms. Standard operating procedures in their most basic form represent cognitive structures of learning. Given the global competitive environment, most firms must also unlearn routines and old behaviors and be willing to investigate their intelligence gathering and processing to see if it is still reliable and performing well. For example, retailers, such as Kroger, have obtained years of efficiency gains that allowed them to digest much higher pandemic sales volume—both in-store and online. This firm evidences cognitive structures of learning at work. Simultaneously, the retailer earned profits from its media business that makes money from ad dollars from online sales.

What is poorly understood outside the literature is the difficulty that firms have managing and deciphering changes in their environment whether they are regulatory, market-driven, or technological in nature. While the threats can be quite meaningful in of themselves, the steeper challenge for many lies with how to interpret or how to make sense of what these changes truly engender for the firm. Making strategic choices in such bumpy waters mandates that senior leadership match those choices to their understanding of the environment in which they find themselves. Individuals possess multiple frames from which they can pull at any given time. If such multiple frames do exist simultaneously, then how are such frames adopted within a management group, tasked with makes strategic choices, where there is a multiplication of such frames at work? Is there a frame or schema that dominates over the others? For Costco, its senior leadership adopted a prevailing frame that interpreted some of the pandemic changes early, seen in its strong sales of fresh foods while keeping up labor productivity and spoilage down.

It is helpful to fill this void by advocating a position that classifies these moments of multiple frames as "framing contests" where each actor seeks to engage others in adopting his frame through lobbying or mobilizing others (Martin, 2017). This is a dynamic, purposive view of framing. While this is clearly a perspective based on political processes at work within a firm, its value lies in unmasking how framing in strategy-making actually involves individuals struggling in marketing their own particular frame, which is too, intertwined with pushing their own particular political interests on behalf of the firm (Hänggli & Kriesi, 2012). For example, management at Viacom CBS is struggling with how much to spend on its new streaming service so as to attract new subscribers, but still maintain its traditional TV business. This suggests managers are vying to promote their own frame to be used in strategy-making.

This view also draws out of the social movement research above, who underscored early that framing was more than the use of ordinary tools, but also "schemata of interpretation" which allowed managers to engage in sensemaking in rather ambiguous and unpredictable environments. Firms that experience inertia, such as the movie theatre chains outlined above, may suggest that a prevailing frame could not be adopted in the contest over meanings or perhaps an existing frame was hardwired in such that newer frames could not compete or be accepted as legitimate, and the result is unresolved issues or deferred decisions. It could also be that a frame is so deeply embedded within the firm with a set of interests allied with it that the frame remains as it is, which represents a consensus of what the strategy of the firm is.

CONCLUSION

This chapter has sought to understand how cognitive frames or schemata influence organizational strategy making, especially in times of pandemics. Such understanding is essential for unraveling how managers scan, read, and interpret ambiguous data coming into the firm from an unpredictable, ever-changing, threatening, competitive arena. Understanding how managers frame information improves decision-making. Similarly, it is quite clear from the literature that it is the management group that constructs meaning within a firm. Also, framing is directly relatable to the firm's performance. When one considers the fortunes of a firm such as Kodak, who failed to correctly interpret the ambiguous signals of the market that its chief product, film, was in the midst of being transformed into digital imaging, this enlightens how framing truly matters for a firm's well-being.

Similarly, firms can change their knowledge structures or frames of reference. There were framing contests at work within the walls of the firm that were just as intense and passionate as the battles in the marketplace. What is interesting is that frame adoption or realignment represent collective efforts at meaning making. It is hardly an individual's effort normally. This idea of struggles within the firm of how to interpret and how to respond to perceived threats helps with deciphering why some firms do what they do and that knowledge structures do change potentially with each hard-fought contest. Lastly, it is clear that CEOs do surveil their environment with the frames or schemata they have, which serve as both constraints and resources to them. The strategic choices that they make couple together both diagnostic and prognostic elements. It is in this action of making choices that shows evidence of knowledge structures, frames of reference, mental scripts, or schemata at work that define what the firm is, what it will do, and when it will do it.

REFERENCES

Berger, P. L., & Luckmann, T. (1966). *The social construction of reality: A treatise in the sociology of knowledge.* Doubleday.

Christensen, C., & Raynor, M. (2003). *The innovator's solution*. Harvard Business School Press.

Daft, R., & Weick, K. (1984). Toward a model of organizations as interpretation systems. *The Academy of Management Review, 9*(2), 284–295. http://www.jstor.org.ezproxy.fiu.edu/stable/258441

Fiss, P., & Zajac, E. (2006). The symbolic management of strategic change: Sensegiving via framing and decoupling. *The Academy of Management Journal, 49*(6), 1173–1193. http://www.jstor.org.ezproxy.fiu.edu/stable/20159826

Gasparro, A., & Terlep, S. (2021). These brands think working from home is here to stay. *The Wall Street Journal.* https://www.wsj.com/articles/consumer-brands-bet-working-from-home-is-here-to-stay-11609065000?mod=Searchresults_pos1&page=1

Hänggli, R. (2020). Frame construction for media input (strategic framing choices). In *The origin of dialogue in the news media* (pp. 67–92). Palgrave Macmillan. https://doi.org/10.1007/978-3-030-26582-3_4

Hänggli, R., & Kriesi, H. (2012). Frame construction and frame promotion (strategic framing choices). *American Behavioral Scientist, 56*(3), 260–278. https://doi.org/10.1177/0002764211426325

Martin, B. H. (2017). Unsticking the status quo: Strategic framing effects on managerial mindset, status quo bias and systematic resistance to change. *Management Research Review, 40*(2), 122–141. https://doi.org/10.1108/MRR-08-2015-0183

Mims, C. (2021). Amazon's new CEO, Andy Jassy, can either help workers and sellers—Or automate them away. *The Wall Street Journal,* https://www.wsj.com/articles/amazons-new-ceo-can-either-help-workers-and-sellers-or-automate-them-away-11612587602?mod=Searchresults_pos13&page=1

Nassauer, S. (2021). Walmart sales growth helped by stimulus. *The Wall Street Journal.* https://www.wsj.com/articles/walmart-sales-rise-even-as-pandemic-wanes-11621338667?mod=Searchresults_pos1&page=1

Sandberg, J., & Tsoukas, H. (2015). Making sense of the sensemaking perspective: Its constituents, limitations, and opportunities for further development. *Journal of Organizational Behavior, 36*(S1), S6–S32. https://doi.org/10.1002/job.1937

Weick, K. (1995). *Sensemaking in organizations*. SAGE.

CHAPTER 10

JOB SEARCH FOR THE LONG-TERM UNEMPLOYED

A Practical Approach for Practitioners

Robert H. Tiell and S. Charles Malka

While the pandemic hit harshly millions who lost their jobs, it is affecting particularly hard the long-term job seekers, a sizable group that exceeded four million in early 2021. Despite their numbers, the long-term unemployed (LTU) have historically attracted little programmatic attention from policy makers and practitioners in the field. We refer to the paucity of interest that characterized the treatment of the LTU in an earlier work (Malka & Tiell, 2016), as well as in another chapter of this book. Surveys show for example that the percentage of LTU in February 2021 is comparable to the peak long-term unemployed percentage that we saw back in 2010 (Sharone, 2021).

This low interest is surprising given that unemployment affects other related policy issues that tend to garner a heightened public discourse. Among such issues are the extension of unemployment benefits, efforts to raise the minimum wage, and earning disparities (Manning, 2021; Rampell, 2020). Equally perplexing, the abundance of studies focusing on

Back to a New Normal: In Search of Stability in an Era of Pandemic Disruption—Insight From Practitioners and Academics, pp. 133–147

unemployment as a construct provide only a few practical cases that apply empirical knowledge for the design and development of intervention programs. A decade ago, Katz (2010) could name only a handful of community-based employment programs that connect job seekers with local and regional employers. Years later, a survey of directors of career and employment service providers from 30 major cities in the U.S. found no documented programs that specifically targeted the long-term unemployed for intervention purposes (Malka & Tiell, 2016).

Unlike the meager attention given by policy makers and practitioners to the unemployed, scholars have studied unemployment for quite some time. An emerging broad theme is that the unemployed experience a deepening loss of self-worth, which in turn often generates a downward psychological cycle infused with emotional reactions including anxiety, depression and despair. But while challenges faced by the LTU parallel those faced by any unemployed person, the LTU arguably face additional unique and onerous challenges. The LTU faces the erosion of work-related skills that occurs in the aftermath of job loss with the passing of time.

Just as critical is the increasing stigma and potential employment discrimination encountered simply by virtue of being out of work for an extended period, as some employers do in fact discriminate against the LTU (Leubsdorf, 2014). Considering these dynamics, it should come as no surprise that many of these individuals ultimately feel increasingly helpless, vulnerable, and resource-depleted as time passes.

Job search and job readiness training programs must adapt their approach to address the needs of this challenged population. At the core of this approach is the belief that meaningful interventions must address a person's present psychological status, which are typically not addressed in the myriad job search workshops and programs created to help the long-term job seeker (Sharone, 2014). Our approach asserts the important role that psychological-emotional factors play as barriers for the LTU, as well as the critical role that traditional-technical job search factors also play in reaching reemployment outcomes. For instance, how well the LTU integrates a specific set of actions such as developing resume writing and interviewing skills, networking and social media utilization, understanding workforce trends, and various job search techniques should make a substantial difference in the success of one's job search.

Similarly, the importance of helping individuals align themselves with the specifications and qualifications of the job being sought cannot be understated. To proceed otherwise is missing an important piece and sets a job seeker up for failure. Therefore, to create a truly effective job search delivery system for the members of this unique LTU population, traditional-technical job search practices are necessary but insufficient. They must be combined with best practices for managing the less traditional but critically important psychological variables that impede job search success, but which are historically ignored when developing job search best practices.

PREVAILING JOB SEARCH PRACTICES ARE INSUFFICIENT

Sharone (2014) examined what he believes occur in most intervention programs designed for the unemployed. Assessing current job search practices among a U.S. West coast population, he identified dominant and prevailing characteristics and asserted that these job search practices create a marked tendency among the unemployed to view themselves as somehow flawed and tend toward self-blame rendering them more likely to remain jobless over time. Sharone's contribution appears valuable for it provides a snapshot of practices and procedures utilized by job search practitioners and providers. Furthermore, it highlights shortcomings that must be overcome when considering future delivery models. According to Sharone, the prevailing American job search model has several key characteristics:

- The model grew out of the self-help industry which spawned a plethora of job search books and materials.
- Current job search practice is further predicated on a 'chemistry game' which requires that the job seeker put their personality on the line, establish rapport, and quickly draw a strong personal connection to the interviewer/recruiter or otherwise risk losing out. Job search practices predicated on the chemistry game may pay dividends and generate results in the earlier stages of one's job search but may not be sustainable for the longer haul.
- Job search practice tends to focus on self, personal attributes and likeability as opposed to skills, core job specifications, and how well one's qualifications align with a position's specific job requirements.
- Considerable emphasis is put on the overall quality of one's job search documents, especially, the resume and cover letter. The quality of these documents influences one's probability for landing a job.
- Job seekers are urged to strategize and set employment goals driven primarily by their passion and what they view as their dream job.

- Job search success hinges pretty much on oneself. Market driven forces that many view as outside one's personal control play a less significant role in job search workshop practice.

Due to the inordinate emphasis on the internal self as opposed to external factors, the job seeker will likely not be prompted to attend to, or sufficiently incorporate, structural changes in the economy, industry trends, labor market information, business research, employer perceptions, and other external market driven realities potentially critical for a truly effective job search. Furthermore, the above set of practices tend to ultimately lead the job seeker down a path toward self-blame with many of its attendant negative consequences. These observations highlight the important role that one's view of oneself plays in job search success. The longer one goes without desired employment, the greater the likelihood the individual will convert to long-term unemployment and experience negative reactions ranging from frustration and anxiety to depression and perhaps even despair.

Because these internal, psychological, behavioral health features are viewed as integral to job search success, the authors created a new delivery model to address these relevant behavioral health factors, in addition to traditional job search methods and techniques. In this vein, we created a program using a holistic service delivery model that incorporates both traditional job-search elements and nontraditional behavioral health interventions for helping the LTU.

Given the scale and challenges of our target population and the meager number of documented intervention programs, a pilot study was initially carried out with a small group of LTUs to determine the impact of a unique delivery model on participants' job search success and return to the workforce. Building on existing cognitive theories, the program intervention targeted the unique, diverse needs of the LTU. The following section briefly describes some of the theories undergirding our program, the delivery model structure, details of the workshop and lessons learned. Recommendations for the future are also discussed.

A NEW DELIVERY MODEL: THEORETICAL UNDERPINNINGS

This section provides a brief synopsis of relevant practical applications of empirical findings and highlights the contribution cognitive theories have had on the development of our model. Development of our delivery model was influenced by empirical works that focused on job search antecedents, efficacy, and job search success (Malka & Tiell, 2016; Sharone, 2014; Wanberg et al., 2010). Our workshop's curriculum was also shaped by additional theories such as adult learning theory (Knowles, 1984), Peter's personal branding principles (Peters, 1999), and Krumboltz' happenstance learning theory (Krumboltz, 2009).

Briefly stated, one principle embedded in adult learning theory which was incorporated greatly into the delivery model is the principle of experiential learning (Knowles, 1984). Experiential learning suggests that many people learn best by doing. This in turn extends to the notion that, beyond didactic methods, the opportunity for practical application of material further facilitates the job search learning process. Peter's personal branding principles (Peters, 1999) are generally credited with drawing attention to the importance of personal branding—self-packaging and self-marketing—with a focus on one's unique value proposition. Krumboltz's happenstance learning theory posits that chance events over the course of one's life can have positive or negative impact depending on how it is viewed. Moreover, unpredictable events or conditions including LTU can greatly influence one's life including work related decisions (Krumboltz, 2009).

Social cognitive theory also lies at the heart of many works that deal with job search intent and behavior. Social cognitive theory asserts that observational learning and modeling also can shape effective job search behavior (Bandura, 1989). One related perspective, self-regulation theory, argues that job search begins with an employment goal followed by self-regulating actions (Lahuis, 2005). Building on this perspective, an important part of our delivery model was setting personal employment goals followed by concrete regulating actions. Group and individual assignments allowed for customization of self-regulating actions and encouraged group feedback. Complementing this process, one session was devoted to clarifying job search attitudes and self-efficacy, both determinants of job search intensity, which in turn affects the frequency and scope of specific job search behavior.

An additional determinant of subsequent job search behavior is job search progress. Self-regulation theory posits that individuals adjust their effort given the perception of their progress toward a set goal (Bandura, 1989). Building on the latter, the intervention model incorporated brief surveys designed to assess the level of perceived progress after each session as reported by participants. Monitoring progress allowed for a better alignment of each participant with a customized employment action plan. Final progress reports were completed 90-day postintervention to assess the overall impact of workshops on participants job search success.

Another critical aspect of the model involved dissemination and assessment of job market information. Lopez-Kidwell et al. (2013) reported that active job seekers lower their job search uncertainties as they gain access to more and better job market information. The authors suggested that job seekers derive their most useful job search information from other individuals with whom they are connected. The group format used for each workshop session was designed to encourage a continuous peer information exchange, and act as a social network extension. The authors were also cognizant of social comparison theory's premise (Festinger, 1954) that emphasizes the influence of peers and referent others on an individual's own behavior. Consequently, it was assumed that job seekers will tend to adopt job search levels like those of their network peers, more so in situations of uncertainty.

Finally, a critical part of this program aimed at identifying and enhancing psychological resilience of participants who experienced prolonged job loss and job search setback. While continued job seeking behavior is enhanced by prior success, such behavior is undermined by setbacks. Negative effects of setbacks can be ameliorated by behavioral inoculation, promoting trust and providing continued social support. Among them are having unemployed individuals anticipate situations in which setbacks or relapses are likely, generating alternative methods for overcoming dysfunctional responses to setbacks, and acquiring skills needed to cope with such setbacks. Some of the rehearsed scenarios during program sessions followed these guidelines closely. In addition, several workshop sessions addressed cognitive resilience and setback management by focusing on emotions and mind set, as well as stress management and reframing behaviors via success stories.

CONSIDERING A FEW GUIDING PRINCIPLES

Observing members of our target population up close, many with advanced degrees and impressive credentials, it was surmised that in addition to a lack of technical aspects of job search, LTU more often contributes to adverse psychological consequences. This ultimately creates adverse behavioral health effects, which in turn results in persistent and prolonged unemployment. Thus, an effective job search intervention for the LTU must address both traditional-technical job search methods and the nontraditional behavioral health interventions heretofore largely ignored. Our psychoeducational delivery model presented here combines both customary technical job search techniques and typically neglected behavioral health techniques. With that operational framework in mind, a series of sessions were tailored specifically to members of this vulnerable LTU group.

Beyond continuation of traditional job search strategies, the goal of the workshop series was essentially twofold. Firstly, to give participants the knowledge and ability to work through the job search process with sharpened clarity and insight, thereby increasing gainful employment prospects. Secondly, to give participants the opportunity to address psychoemotional challenges induced by job search stress and develop behavioral health techniques to reinstall confidence and thereby accelerate effective job search behaviors.

Based on both research and practice, certain principles guided our thinking and approach in working with the LTU:

- The LTU are a distinct population a subset of the more traditional unemployed, and a subset that is commonly beset with many unique challenges that can, if not careful, compound and prolong their length of unemployment.
- The LTU's challenges are primarily linked to the deepening psychological and behavioral health domain, and behavioral health barriers can thereby readily surface and impede success.
- Traditional job search techniques and methods that are typically used and emphasized in unemployed group workshop formats are necessary, but insufficient.
- A unique approach created for this workshop revolved around the behavioral health and cognitive-psychological realm, which in turn also draws from the field of positive psychology (Seligman, 2006), adult learning theory and practice, a psychoeducational perspective, and a personal branding focus.

THE DELIVERY MODEL'S CONTEXT AND DYNAMICS

The community-based career services organization that was tasked with the delivery of our model provided a unique context for executing the kind of workshops intended for this program.

First, the organization employed an interdisciplinary staff with a diverse set of skills and experience that promote a more eclectic and effective workshop experience for participants. In addition, the organization engaged in psychometric evaluation and utilized various tools to assess change and progress. The combination of skilled staff and effective instrumentation helped workshop participants gain insight regarding their personal strengths and how their assets could be leveraged for employment search purposes. Metrics were also used to assess forces that present barriers to employment, such as interview anxiety.

Second, many LTUs have at least one or two key what we term 'stuck' related issues which leave them at an impasse in their job search. These 'stuck' factors can easily delay or undercut one's job search. We built on principles of positive psychology in addressing and ameliorating participants' 'stuck' areas as a way for releasing positive energy and progress. The field of positive psychology influenced the way in which this workshop was designed and delivered. Psychology as a discipline, particularly the clinical psychology specialty, has historically focused on and assessed one's problems in more pathological terms. Contrary to this traditional view, positive psychology is a branch of psychology which views the individual in terms of strengths and assets rather than in terms of one's weaknesses or deficits (Seligman, 2006).

Third, various features and strands linked to the positive psychology movement were introduced into the workshops' curriculum. This included research around mind-body connections, personal strengths, self-efficacy, locus of control, emotional-social intelligence, success stories, and other topics relevant to how the cognitive framework can affect job search. In many respects, the concept of self-efficacy has special relevance for the topic of LTU. Among other things, self-efficacy speaks to confidence, learned optimism, assertiveness, and initiative-taking behavior, all of which are important for being able to mount and sustain a challenging job search.

Finally, the workshops embraced experiential approaches to new learning, including participant feedback. The opportunity to practice and apply the material participants were introduced to, urged to learn, and advised to internalize was also instrumental to the success of each workshop.

Another fact that carried importance for our target workshop participants was the rethinking of careers and jobs in much less traditional ways. Todays' job seekers face a vastly different job market compared to past generations. For example, approximately a third of the contemporary workforce now consists of contingent workers—individuals who are freelance, temporary, project-driven, and untethered to a specific employer. Trends such as this become a critical reality test for workshop participants. Toward this end, some of Peters' (1999) personal branding principles, as well as Krumboltz's (2009) happenstance learning theory, were incorporated as a means of encouraging participants to assert self-control, take initiative and action, embrace self-marketing, and adopt a personal branding frame of mind.

A NEW DELIVERY MODEL: WORKSHOP SESSIONS

The workshops' sessions and content are shown in Table 10.1. The selected sessions and their sequence were determined largely by several criteria that included the research literature, traditional nuts and bolts of

Table 10.1

Workshop Modules

Session 1	Session 2
• Registration • Welcome and introductions: rating measures • Creating a common language • Understanding ourselves • Assessment feedback • Mind-body connections: the role stress and anxiety play • Employment search skills • Homework	• Review and recap of Session 1 • Identifying your "stuck" area • Understanding your mind set and emotions • Stress and anxiety management • Benefits of relaxation techniques • Job search skills & Self-efficacy • Success stories • Marketing yourself: Creating your commercial • Networking and social media • Homework
Session 3	**Session 4**
• Review and recap of Session 2 • Continued work on "stuck" clusters • Job search skills and self-efficacy extended • Gearing up both locus of control & emotional/social intelligence • Job search clarity • Small group breakouts and opportunity for behavioral rehearsal • Bottom line impact • Homework	• Review and recap Session 3 • Facilitator feedback • Practicing and applying learned techniques, behaviors, and strategies • Integrating and fine tuning technical and behavioral employment action plan • Continue breakouts for individualizing purposes • Participant commitment and next steps • Final integrating comments and wrap-up • Postworkshop evaluation

job search content and techniques, prevailing workshop delivery practice, workshop facilitators, job search best practices, and the intent to incorporate a balance of traditional and behavioral help techniques. An entire set of new behavioral health content that historically had not been incorporated into job search workshops was woven into our service delivery model. This was considered critical in dealing with various psychodynamic issues pertinent to the target LTU population.

Thus, workshops included sessions that addressed topics such as: (a) assessment measures and feedback to help participants gauge status and progress, (b) review of traditional job search materials and methods, (c) exploration of the role behavioral health features customarily play in job searches typical of the LTU, (d) examination of factors that tend to prompt the LTU to get emotionally stuck, and (e) ultimately the creation of a more holistic, psychology healthy and effective employment action plan.

Sessions also included sections on technical skills such as social media, elevator pitch, answering tough interview questions, and resume critique. However, much time was also dedicated toward helping participants understand their psychoemotional reactions to job search setback and frustration while also learning how to manage these feelings and emotions in constructive ways. Techniques such as relaxation, imagery, and cognitive reframing were used to relieve stress and anxiety (Hope et al., 2010). A section on feelings, core emotions, and "I Messages" helped participants verbalize how they can constructively express and display their feelings in the face of frustration and anger.

CONSIDERATION OF MEASURES USED

Three behavioral assessments, completed by participants prior to beginning of each workshop, were used as tools for self-reflection and processing throughout each workshop. These metrics included Career Strengths Finder, Locus of Control, and the EQ Quick Scan. Strengths Finder assists each participant in identifying major strengths to be leveraged for job search purposes (Rath, 2007). Locus of Control helps participants gauge personal control (i.e., the extent to which the participant believes he/she can shape positive job search outcomes) (Hill, 2013). The EQ Quick Scan identifies a participant's emotional intelligence (EQ) and the ways EQ can be enacted to cope with the relational demands of a job search, for example networking and negotiation (Bradberry & Greaves, 2009).

These metrics all connect well with the positive psychology movement. Results of these assessments were reviewed and explained to each workshop participant, with feedback given to promote optimal understanding of how results can impact one's job search as the employment journey ensues. Ultimately, participants left the program with a better understanding of themselves and their personal assets, techniques to manage their feelings, employment tips and strategies and a written employment action plan.

Six different metrics were used throughout and after this workshop series to measure progress, impact and outcomes. The metrics measuring anxiety, job search clarity, anxiety in selection interviewing, and the five-factor metric were adopted from validated scales used in other works. The postevaluation and postintervention employment appraisal survey was developed by the delivery organization:

- *Anxiety.* Workshop participants were surveyed weekly on their general anxiety level. Based on the Depression and Anxiety Stress Scale (Lovibond & Lovibond, 1995), participants were asked to rate their recently experienced level of anxiety. The scale was administered after each workshop session for a total of four administrations per participant.

- *Job Search Clarity.* Participants were surveyed on their job search clarity using a scale adapted from the one developed by Cote, Saks, and Zikic (2006). This one-item measure asks participants to rate their current level of clarity and focus as they reflect on their job search effort. This metric was administered pre- and postworkshop intervention.
- *Measure of Anxiety in Selection Interviewing.* The Measure of Anxiety in Selection Interviews is a metric adapted from McCarthy and Goffin (2004) which examines the level of anxiety one brings to job interviews. The measure was administered pre- and postworkshop.
- *Five-Factor Metric.* A five-factor metric was administered to participants who rated their traits across various job search features, such as one's level of self-confidence in mounting a job search, and reduced anxiety in managing the job search process. The Five factor metric was administered pre and post workshop.
- *Postevaluation Form.* Upon completion, workshop participants were asked for their feedback on a 15-item questionnaire, rating their satisfaction with specific workshop components. Items included resume development, interviewing, employment action plans, mental barriers, psychological-emotional influences, and confidence level/comfort with various interview situations and their newly acquired and expanded job search strategies.
- *Securing Employment.* The final workshop indicator was whether participants secured employment during or soon after workshop completion. Follow-up contact with participants was conducted to appraise employment status and return to work.

ON THE OVERALL IMPACT OF THE DELIVERY MODEL

Within 3 months of our first workshop completion, 68% of participants found satisfactory full-time positions. This pattern continued with other subsequent workshops carried out by the career service organization advancing ultimately to a 90% employment rate. Our delivery system appears to validate the vast majority of the assertions that were made regarding the delivery model, and the wisdom of incorporating principles from fields like positive psychology and adult learning theory. A key assertion relates to the use of both traditional and nontraditional job search methods. The positive impact that our combined set of interventions had on participants' job search suggested that incorporating traditional and nontraditional job search methods appears fully warranted and necessary. Conducting a job search workshop for the LTU without addressing the behavioral health implications is clearly insufficient.

Undergirding the delivery of nontraditional behavioral health features in the workshop seems to align well with the tenets of positive psychology. Self-efficacy perspectives, as well, flow naturally out of the positive psychology field and appear worthy of consideration when contemplating workshop content. Some of the claims concerning positive psychology, appear relevant to adult learning theory as well.

Building on this principle of experiential learning, workshop participants were provided with the opportunity for practical application of sessions' material that further facilitated the job search learning process. Our experience suggests that behavioral rehearsal and role playing were useful for many workshop participants and are worth also continuing as part of the workshop process.

Another assertion that was validated concerns the use of an interdisciplinary approach as it relates to workshop facilitators. Involving professionals who bring skills and experience across pertinent disciplines allowed the program to address a more diverse array of issues that tend to surface when dealing with the LTU. The workshop involved specialists in the areas of career and workforce development, psychology, the behavioral sciences, and human resources, all of which proved extremely useful when dealing with a challenging population.

Finally, the introduction of workforce information and trends proved extremely beneficial. Our intervention touched on and addressed factors related to the changing economy and workforce trends. Arguably, temporary, contingent, and project-driven work roles have become more common, and this dynamic has significant implications for how future job seekers will need to maneuver and seek employment. Peters (1999) has long advocated for adopting a "brand you" approach to the way job seekers should view themselves, especially for purposes of self-marketing and promotion.

A NEW DELIVERY MODEL: LESSONS LEARNED

Four key lessons that may benefit other practitioners are worth mentioning:

- First, the workshops were developed with the practitioner in mind. The hands-on perspective was supported by a theoretical layer that allowed for viewing the LTU experience from both theoretical and practitioner perspectives (Malka & Tiell, 2016). Blending the two perspectives, added potency to the model with recommendations benefiting both practitioners and the LTU population.

- Second, the psychological and behavioral health component is not only critical for building resiliency and for setback inoculation, but combining it with the traditional-technical job search components as described earlier is necessary.
- Third, toward this end, a delivery system that is interdisciplinary and draws on career and workforce development, behavioral sciences, business and human resource fields allowed the program to be crafted from a holistic perspective and approach. This allows for the LTU experience to be addressed from multiple directions.
- Finally, while the workshops' behavioral health and technical components proved very useful, they are merely only one important piece of our delivery model. Other beneficial components were the assessment tools, participant feedback, behavioral rehearsal opportunities, and overall experiential features associated with the workshop delivery model.

PRACTICAL RECOMMENDATIONS

We firmly believe there is overriding value in utilizing a delivery model that embraces both traditional and nontraditional psychological methods. We encourage practitioners contemplating the design of a delivery model for the LTU to incorporate the following additional recommendations:

- First, recognize the power and influence of employer perceptions. Employer perceptions play a role in exacerbating the barriers face by the LTU. Studies suggest that members of this vulnerable group are half as likely as short-term unemployed to get a call back (Aaronson et al., 2010). Call back rates for otherwise identical resumes fall sharply as unemployment duration lengthens. To land an interview, the LTU must apply to 3.5 times as many jobs compared to the short-term unemployed. Employers may be screening out applicants based on duration of unemployment and thereby miss many qualified applicants.
- Second, help participants create bridging experiences. Our workshops tried to help participants see the benefit of various bridging experiences as a means of easing the transition back into the workplace. Be it volunteer work, internships, trial nonpaid work, brush-up classes, online courses, short-term credentialing, or various

forms of community engagement, bridging or interim-step experiences can enhance one's employability and strengthen job prospects.

- Third, consider occupation and industry sector specific LTU subgroups when conducting future workshops. The participants in our program represented different lines of work, different educational-training backgrounds, and different life experiences. Participants may gain even greater leverage and impact to the extent they can more strongly identify with fellow participants who have more in common in terms of occupational affiliation and educational backgrounds. Hence, they may be able to better mentor or assist a workshop peer.
- Finally, blend in more individualized workshop features. To better accommodate each participant's specific issues and concerns, it is recommended that one-to-one support features be blended into the program. This allows staff to customize each participant's preferred work goals and employment action plan. Although not formally instituted as a part of the pilot workshop format, workshop leaders added brief one-to-one time with each participant to sharpen their employment strategy. However, in many respects, this one-to-one time was insufficient for fully addressing participants' individual needs. Thus, workshops should add some individualized features to heighten workshop success.

AUTHORS' NOTE

This is a modified version of R. Tiell and S. C. Malka (2017), "Job search turnaround: The case of the long-term unemployed—A practitioner's perspective, *Vocational Evaluation and Work Adjustment Association Journal, 41*(1), 40–55. Used and modified with permission.

REFERENCES

Aaronson, D., Mazumder, B., & Schechter, S. (2010). What is behind the rise in long-term unemployment? *Economic Perspectives, Federal Reserve Bank, Chicago, 34*(2), 28–51.

Bandura, A. (1989). Human agency in social cognitive theory. *American Psychologist, 44*, 1175–1184.

Bradberry, T., & Greaves, J. (2009). *Emotional Intelligence; 2.0*. San Diego, CA: Talent Smart.

Cote, S., Sakes, A. M., & Zikic, J. (2006). Trait affect and job search outcomes. *Journal of Vocational Behavior, 68*(2), 233–252.

Festinger, L. (1954). A theory of social comparison processes. *Human Relations, 7*, 117–140.

Hill, R. (2013). *Teaching internal locus of control: A positive psychological approach*. Beach Haven, NJ: Will Power Press.

Hope, D. A., Burns, J. A., Hyes, S. A., Herbert, J. D., & Warner, M. D. (2010). Automatic thoughts and cognitive restructuring in cognitive behavioral group therapy for social anxiety disorder. *Cognitive Therapy Research, 34*, 1–12

Katz, F. L. (2010, April). *Long-term unemployment in the great recession*. Testimony for the U.S. Congress Joint Economic Committee.

Knowles, M. (1984). *The adult learner: A neglected species*. Houston, TX: Gulf Publishing.

Krumboltz, J. D. (2009). Happenstance learning theory. *Journal of Career Assessment, 17*(2), 135–154.

Lahuis, D. M. (2005). Individual differences in applicant reactions: A job search perspective. *International Journal of Selection and Assessment, 13*, 150–159.

Leubsdorf, B. (2014, January 28). Obama tries new tack for long-term jobless. *Wall Street Journal*, B2. Retrieved from www.wsj.com/public/page/archive-2014-1-28.html

Lopez-Kidwell, V., Grosser, J. T., Dineen, R. B., & Borgatti, P. S. (2013). What matters when: A multistage model and empirical examination of job search effort. *Academy of Management Journal, 56*(6), 1655–1678.

Lovibond, P.F., & Lovibond, S. H. (1995). The structure of the negative emotional states: Comparison of the Depression Anxiety Stress Scale (DASS) with the Beck Depression and Anxiety Inventories. *Behavior Research and Therapy, 33*, 335–343.

Malka, S., & Tiell, R. (2016). Job search turnaround and the long term unemployed: An exploratory framework and a contingency model. *Vocational Evaluation and Career Assessment Professionals Journal, 11*(1), 9–26.

Manning, A. (2021). The Elusive Employment Effect of the Minimum Wage. *Journal of Economic Perspectives, 35*(1), 3–26.

McCarthy, J., & Goffin, R. (2004). Measuring job interview anxiety: Beyond weak and sweaty palms. *Personnel Psychology*, 57, 607–637.

Peters, T. (1999). *Brand You 50*. New-York, NY: Alfred A. Knopf.

Rampell, C. (2020; August 3). The myth of unemployment benefits depressing work. *The Washington Post*, p.D4.

Rath, T. (2007). *Strengths Finder*. New-York, NY: Gallup Press.

Seligman, M. (2006). *Learned optimism: How to change your mind and your life*. New York, NY: Vintage Books.

Sharone, O. (2021, March 18). A Crisis of long-term unemployment is looming in the U.S., *Harvard Business Review*.

Sharone, O. (2014). *Flawed system-flawed self: Job searching and unemployed experiences*. Chicago, IL: University of Chicago Press.

Wanberg, C. R., Zhu, J., & van Hooft, E. A. J. (2010). The job search grind: Perceived progress, self-reactions, and self-regulation of search effort. *Academy of Management Journal, 53*(4), 788–807.

CHAPTER 11

BUSINESS SUSTAINABILITY DURING A PANDEMIC

Practical Steps to Succession Planning

Orville Blackman

The size of the economic fall-out from COVID 19 is still being assessed. As businesses—small and large—begin to regroup their employees who have been largely working remotely, they are still making calculations about when it is safe to return to work at the office. The impact on business was swift and uncalculated. Organizations were driven into unplanned change as employees scrambled to carry on business as usual, while almost nothing in the world was "as usual."

As businesses begin to regroup, we are reflecting on some of the lessons learned from the pandemic. One of the lessons is that there should be a greater urgency to plan for business continuation should the key leaders in the organizations become incapacitated and not be able to lead. The need for active succession planning rises in importance as we review the statistics of those who were most severely affected by the pandemic—those age 60 and above which includes the senior leadership of several organizations.

COVID-19 is a global pandemic that has a debilitating effect on business globally. A report from the World Bank at the height of the pandemic

Back to a New Normal: In Search of Stability in an Era of Pandemic Disruption—Insight From Practitioners and Academics, pp. 149–160

in October 2020 encapsulated the debilitating effects of the pandemic on firms in various countries. The data were collected through pulse surveys in participating countries. The findings suggested that firms globally experienced significant declines in sales and experienced reduced access to finance to sustain operations. A substantial number of firms indicated that they were on the brink of insolvency, potentially leading to more unemployment losses and the threat of permanent closure.

The World Bank study indicated that the firms most susceptible to business failure tended to be more prevalent in poorer countries and were typically smaller firms. Smaller firms also tended to face the threat of failure and at the very least falling into arrears with creditors in more advanced countries. For example, 50% of smaller firms in the United States were found to have less than 15 days of buffer cash at the height of the pandemic. When compared, larger firms tended to have approximately 65 days of cover. The overall projections for post pandemic recovery for all firms were less than glowing, with firms likely to struggle to return to normal business operations long after the pandemic subsides (World Bank, 2020).

Similar to the World Bank report, other studies captured grim projections for business sustainability in the United States during the pandemic. A study by Fairlie (2020) of the early effects of COVID-19 on small business owners from April 2020 Current Population Survey microdata found significant declines in business ownership during the pandemic. According to the researcher, there was a significant drop in the number of working business owners between February and April 2020. The number of working business owners estimated to be about 15 million in February 2020, dropped to about 11.7 million by April of the same year. The 22% (3.3 million) loss of business owners was the highest on record. Other statistics showed a dramatic decline in the number of hours leaders worked when the researchers evaluated work hours for two or four days a week. The total number of hours worked by all business owners dropped by 20%. Incorporated businesses were not exempt from the changes. They also recorded a drop of approximately 20% despite the stability associated with incorporated businesses (Fairlie, 2020).

The study also examined patterns across gender, race, and immigrant status revealing alarming findings. The report indicated that African American business owners experienced the largest losses, eliminating 41% of active business owners. The next largest group was immigrant business owners which declined by 36%. Next were Latinx businesses that experienced major losses—approximately 32% of business owners halting activity between February and April 2020. Finally, female business owners also suffered a disproportionate drop of 25%.

The preceding statistics highlight the challenges that business leaders face during the pandemic. The multifaceted disruptions, including the unexpected sickness and death of key business leaders make the case for a review of how businesses plan for sustainability in the midst of crises. Leadership through and beyond crises such as the case with COVID-19 requires careful succession planning, development, and mentorship.

WHAT IS SUCCESSION PLANNING AND WHY IT IS IMPORTANT?

Succession planning is a focused process for keeping talent in the pipeline. It is generally 12–36 months of preparation for leadership in the organization (Society for Human Resource Management [SHRM], n.d.). The process includes identifying critical job skills, knowledge, social relationships, and formal organizational practices, and passing them on to the next generation of workers. This process ensures a seamless pipeline of talent within the organization thereby leading to sustainability in times of crisis (SHRM, n.d.).

The business case for succession planning includes (a) the need to adapt to demographic changes and talent scarcity, (b) identifying skill gaps and training needs that are essential to the future of the organization, (c) retaining institutional knowledge at a time when there is rapid technical and scientific innovation, (d) investing in employees as a retention strategy and (e) securing or replacing highly specialized competencies (SHRM, n.d.). Creating a formal plan to follow these best practices is urgent because of the median age of senior executives in organizations.

A Korn-Ferry (2017) study of the top 1,000 companies globally based on revenue, found that the average age of leaders in the C-Suite is 54. The roles examined were chief executive officer, chief financial officer, chief human resources officer, chief marketing officer, and chief information officer. Approximately one quarter of the labor force will be over 55 by 2026. The number is expected to grow from 35.7 million in 2016 to 42.1 million in 2026 (Collins & Casey, 2017). Job losses associated with the COVID-19 recession may be contributing to the jump in Baby Boomers retiring (Fry, 2020)—many of whom may be from among the senior leadership ranks in organizations. Retirement estimates were about 40% in September 2020 and were expected to continue at similar rates. Turner (n.d.) estimated that among them are leaders—approximately 40% of whom are eligible to retire in 5 years.

Discussion about the age of senior leaders is important in the context of the pandemic because of the disproportionate effect of COVID-19 on older people. The Centers for Disease Control and Prevention (CDC, 2021) reported that 8 of 10 deaths in the United States were among people 65 years old and older. This suggests that of the 33 million people who were affected or the 593, 000 people who died (CDC, 2020), some senior leaders in organizations were likely among those who were either incapacitated or passed away as a result COVID-19.

The unexpected loss of leaders has implications for several businesses as they seek to regroup and reposition for growth. Organizations that did not effectively plan for future leadership are likely to struggle to restart and advance operations with people who were not engaged in shaping the strategic direction of the organizations. Statistics indicate that only 10% of small-medium sized businesses tend to have formal succession plans, 38% have informal plans, and 50% do not have any succession plans (SHRM, n.d.). Reflecting on the business case for succession planning, there is an urgency to engage in succession planning especially in light of the unexpected loss of senior talent in organizations due to crises such as the COVID-19 pandemic.

Leaders have found that the transition from other levels of leadership in the organization to the executive have been rather challenging and requires specific preparation for roles in the C-Suite (SHRM, 2008). As organizations consider succession planning as a strategy to prepare leaders for roles on the executive, they should consider the following factors:

Succession Planning as a Strategy

The organization should articulate succession planning as a strategic objective and provide the necessary resources to implement the strategy in the organization. By "calling out" succession planning in its strategic plan, the organization sends a message to stakeholders that it is serious about creating a pipeline of qualified and ready leaders who will sustain its future leadership. It is important to identify who will champion the initiative, leading with a formal design, accompanied by performance metrics to measure progress.

Using a validated strategic planning framework such as the Balanced Scorecard provides a lens through which we can understand the strategic components of organizations and the competencies required to contribute at the highest levels.

The Balanced Scorecard (see Figure 11.1) recommends that we examine an organization from four different perspectives to help develop objectives, key performance indicators (KPIs), targets, and initiatives relative to those views.

- **Financial (or Stewardship):** views an organization's financial performance and the use of financial resources.

Figure 11.1

Balanced Scoreboard Framework

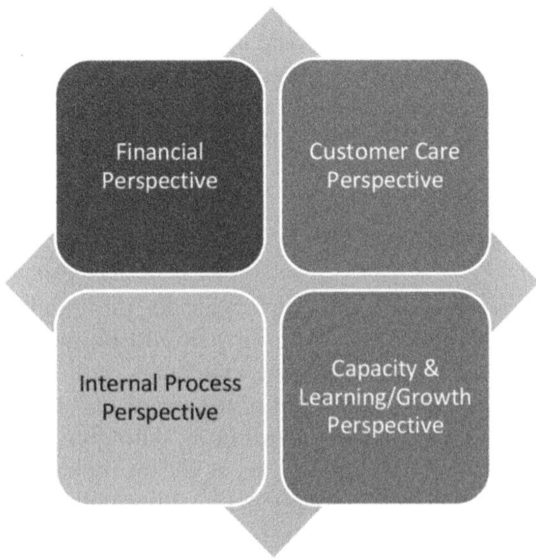

- **Customer/Stakeholder:** views organizational performance from the perspective of the customer or key stakeholders the organization is designed to serve.
- **Internal Process:** views the quality and efficiency of an organization's performance related to the product, services, or other key business processes.
- **Organizational Capacity (or Learning & Growth):** views human capital, infrastructure, technology, culture, and other capacities that are key to breakthrough performance (Balancedscorecard.org).

As a beginning step, organizations should consider what are the mission critical roles in each of the four quadrants of the Balanced Scorecard. Then begin to fill those roles first by identifying candidates who by their knowledge, skills and behaviors exemplify the leadership required in (a) customer care, (b) employee recruitment, selection, development, and retention; (c) operations management including process engineering, and (d) expertise in financial management. While large organizations are likely to hire specialists in these areas, small businesses will likely need to choose well rounded individuals who demonstrate strategic thinking but can also help with implementation at the tactical and operational levels.

The four quadrants of the Balanced Scorecard must be well aligned with the vision, mission, values, and overall strategic objectives of the organization. Without these guiding principles forecasting the next 3–5 years, selection of the next leaders becomes ineffective because talent selections need to be aligned with the organization's strategy. Therefore, before engaging in creating a succession plan, organizations must either engage in strategic planning, or review and validate their strategic plans—from which the objectives of succession planning will emerge.

Measuring Progress

Succession planning programs are typically designed as 2 to 3-year programs (SHRM, 2008). The programs should be governed by formal policy guidelines and have objective outcomes with KPIs. The policy guidelines should require assessment of the needs of the organization as a first step in identifying qualified candidates. The question that needs to be answered is what are the knowledge, skills and behaviors required for leading in the identified leadership roles? Additionally, the policy should include a diversity recruitment directive that ensures that all employees regardless of age, gender, race, national origin, veteran or disability status, sexual orientation, or religious perspective, have fair and equal chances to be considered for the roles. The process must be transparent and guided by standardized rubrics with clear measures that help to preserve fairness and objectivity.

Selecting the Candidate Pool

Selecting candidates for the succession planning program can be fraught with challenges including accusations of favoritism. Candidates should be selected through an objective process that seeks to align the strengths and attributes of the potential candidates with (a) what it takes to be a good leader and (b) the needs of the organization. Chamorrow-Premuzic (2016) in the Harvard Business Review, identified attributes that leaders should look for when evaluating leadership potential. The researcher stated that studies show that emerging leaders tend to be more adjusted, sociable, ambitious, and curious. As much as 53% of the variability in predicting the success of future leaders is explained by these factors.

The preeminent goal of creating a succession planning program is to preserve leadership effectiveness in the organization thereby guaranteeing its sustainability. As organizations plan, they should be cognizant of the measures of leadership effectiveness and create a program that is geared toward effectiveness outcomes. The measures of leadership effectiveness include (a) the positive performance of the team or organization, particularly in relation to other groups or organizations, (b) demonstration of higher levels of integrity which creates a fair and just culture in the team and organization, and (c) exemplifying emotional intelligence which enables them to stay calm under pressure and (d) possessing better people skills.

To begin the selection process, the organizations should assemble a selection committee comprised of seasoned subject matter experts. To reduce selection error and increase confidence in the selection process, the committee should use a triangulation process that includes (a) a tool such as the 9-Box matrix performance grid, (b) one or more behavioral and strengths assessments, and (c) a selection rubric that helps to maintain objectivity and fairness in the process. The selection process should begin with a profile of the ideal candidate for each role that is targeted in the succession plan. Guided by the profiles, managers will recommend suitable candidates from across the organization who meet the criteria stated in the candidate profile.

The nine-box matrix performance grid was created by management consulting firm McKinsey. They created the assessment to help General Electric prioritize investments they were making in their business units (McKinsey & Company, 2008). The nine-box performance grid (see Figure 11.2) contains different areas which measure two factors—performance and potential. Each employee is positioned within a box. The exercise is best done in collaboration with the employee as a part of the performance management process. However, when used for selection of candidates for the succession planning program, the selection committee may use previous performance evaluation documents to map the proposed candidates to the grid. Subsequent conversations with managers and candidates will confirm or disconfirm the candidates' suitability for the succession planning program.

Most businesses need a large number of employees in Boxes 2, 3, 5, and 6 on the performance grid. They demonstrate acceptable levels of performance needed to keep the organization running but are unlikely to reach the highest levels of leadership in the organization. The ideal candidates who are short-listed for the succession planning program should be identified as people who meet the criteria outlined in one of the boxes —6, 8, or 9 in the 9-Box Performance Grid. They demonstrate high potential for growth, tend to be ready to take on the challenge of stretch goals and are among the top talent in the organization.

Employees in the other boxes will require other forms of development that are beyond the scope of the formal succession plan. Those who are mapped to boxes 4 and 7 should have developmental programs that

Figure 11.2

The Nine-Box Performance Grid

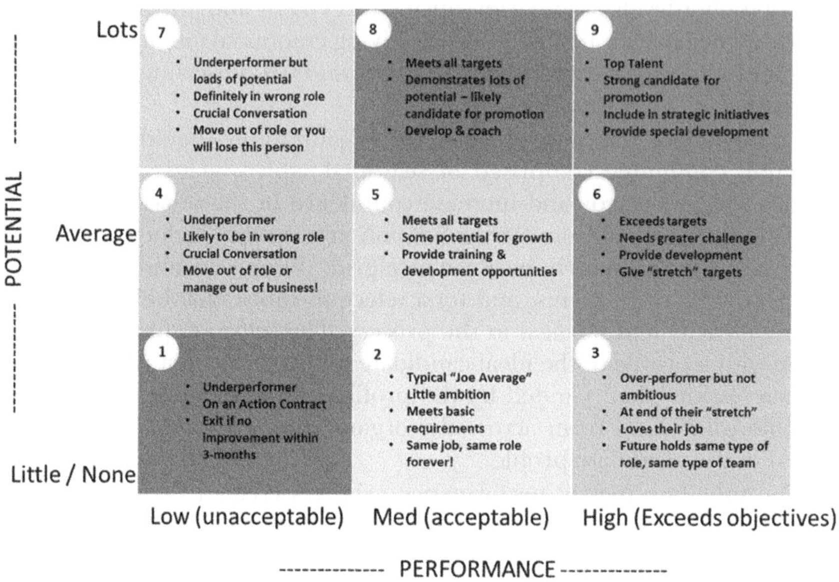

Source: The Balanced Scorecard Institute (n.d.).

move them from under performance to "meets goals" in the short term. Should they fail to progress, they should be subsequently mapped to box 1, where the employees should be coached out of the organization.

The second step in the triangulation process is having the short-listed candidates complete behavioral and strengths assessments. These assessments help to identify the attributes identified for emerging leaders as described by Chamorro-Premuzic (2016). There are more than 100 valid behavioral and cognitive assessments including Wiley's DiSC Product, TotalSDI, PXT Select, Predictive Index, Booth's 360 leadership emotional Intelligence, and Clifton Strengths—formerly StrengthsFinder, that can help narrow the candidates to those whose assessments validate the candidates' suitability for leadership in the organization. The assessments will be reviewed in the context of the candidates' profile to confirm that the candidate has the attributes to successfully complete the succession plan program and ultimately become an effective leader.

The third step in the selection process is to interview short-listed candidates. The selection committee should develop an objective interview protocol that is comprised of open-ended questions about the employee's goals and aspirations, his/her experiences that make her a good leadership candidate, and their willingness and availability to complete an intensive succession planning program.

The final group of succession planning candidates should be selected based on the organization's ability to provide a solid developmental program that includes executive leadership education and mentorship by a suitable senior leader who can help to prepare the candidate for success. The design or selection of an executive leadership program should be guided by the organization's needs based on the mission, vision and values, the anticipated talent gaps that they are preparing to fill, and the program's ability to prepare the leaders to meet the needs of the organization. Leaders should carefully scrutinize the stated outcomes of the executive education programs before investing in a year-long training for each of the succession planning candidates.

Mentorship Program

Having selected the candidates who will participate in the succession planning program, they should be required to complete a yearlong executive management program followed by a year of mentorship with one of the senior leaders in their career streams. The leaders will assist in developing career pathways within the streams. For example, a person with a Finance background who completes the executive development program may select a pathway toward management or corporate finance. This individual will be paired with a senior Finance professional who will help to align leadership skills of the mentee to the intended career pathway.

The American Psychological Association (2006) defined a mentor as a person who can help develop a mentee. Mentors have two functions, (a) the mentor acts as a coach and provides career and professional development. He/she is an advisor on how to improve career performance; (b) The mentor also has a psychosocial function, acting as a role model and support system for the mentee. The functions combined helps to provide lessons on professional growth and general work-life balance. The mentorship relationships can be formal or informal.

Succession planning programs should seek to develop formal mentoring relationships with clear measures and outcomes. This will facilitate more structure and make it easier to measure progress. In the formal mentorship program, the mentors and mentees will collaborate for a 12-month period with the minimum of one meeting per month. The mentor will help to prepare the candidates for strategic leadership roles. They will be focused on the organization's strategic objectives and will learn how to interpret strategy and develop tactics and operational guidelines.

They will also engage in developing best practice in effective leadership based on the characteristics of effective leaders identified earlier by Chamorrow-Premuzic (2016).

Selecting Mentors and Paring With Mentees

The mentors will be selected from among the senior leaders in the organization. For consistency, the selections committee should use the same selection tools that they used with selecting the succession planning candidates with the selection of mentors. Several of the behavioral assessment tools that were identified earlier provide matching opportunities between the candidate and potential mentors. For example, two individuals with two different profiles may be matched because of the future roles they are likely to play. The assessment tools facilitate the pairing of the mentor and mentee profiles and make recommendations on how to best interact with each other. These features in the various assessments use algorithms to help identify similarities and differences in communication styles and makes recommendations on possible pitfalls to be avoided as the mentor and mentee interacts.

Once the candidate has completed the two year leadership training and mentorship programs, he/she should be ready to take on more responsibility in the organization. Whether there is an opening for his/her expertise, the organization should find ways to engage the newly prepared "leader-in-waiting" in leading the organization. There may be projects that the candidates can manage within their fields both to add value and to retain the talent that has been trained and developed for the organization.

Conclusion

The COVID 19 pandemic thrust unplanned changed on millions of organizations across the globe. The unexpected loss of leadership due to death or incapacitation has raised the level of urgency for preparing the next generation of leaders for organizations of all sizes and types. It is important that organizations use objective methods and validated instruments and processes to select and develop the next generation of leaders. The candidates who are selected for a succession planning program should be those who show the greatest promise to be effective leaders in their organizations.

Following a rigorous assessment and selection process, those who are matched based on the stipulated criteria will receive executive leadership development and mentorship with a senior leader. By establishing a formal mentoring program, the organization is better positioned to develop clear outcomes and measure progress in developing the next generation of leaders in the organization. At the conclusion of the program, those candidates who successfully complete the preparation will participate in executive level leadership—if only at the project level, until permanent positions become open for them.

REFERENCES

American Psychological Association. (2006). *Introduction to mentoring: A guide for mentor and mentees.* https://www.apa.org/education/grad/intro-mentoring.pdf

Balanced Scorecard Institute. (n.d.). *The balanced scorecard framework.* https://balancedscorecard.org/

Center for Disease Control and Prevention. (2021, May 14). *COVID-19.* https://www.cdc.gov/coronavirus/2019-ncov/need-extra-precautions/older-adults.html

Center for Disease Control and Prevention. (n.d.). https://www.cdc.gov/coronavirus/2019-nCoV/index.html

Chamorro-Premuzic, T. (2016). Assessing performance: What science tell us about leadership potential. *Harvard Business Review.* https://hbr.org/2016/09/what-science-tells-us-about-leadership-potential

Collins, S., & Casey, R. (2017). *America's aging workforce: Opportunities and challenges.* Report prepared for the Special Committee on Aging, U. S. Senate.

McKinsey & Company. (2008, September 1). Enduring Ideas: The GE–McKinsey nine box matrix. *McKinsey Quarterly.* https://www.mckinsey.com/ business-functions/strategy-and-corporate-finance/our-insights/enduring-ideas-the-ge-and-mckinsey-nine-box-matrix

Fairlie, R. (2020). The impact of COVID-19 on small business owners: Evidence form the first three months after wide-spread social distancing restrictions. *Journal of Economic Management and Strategy.* https://doi.org/10.1111/jems.12400

Fry, R. (2020, November 9). *The pace of boomer retirements has accelerated in the past year.* Pew Research Center.

Korn-Ferry. (2017). *Age and tenure in the C-Suite.* https://www.kornferry.com/about-us/press/age-and-tenure-in-the-c-suite-korn-ferry-institute-study-reveals-trends-by-title-and-industry

SHRM. (2008). *Leadership competencies.* https://www.shrm.org/resourcesandtools/hr-topics/behavioral-competencies/leadership-and-navigation/pages/leadershipcompetencies.aspx

SHRM. (n.d.). *Engaging in succession planning.* https://www.shrm.org/resourcesandtools/tools-and-samples/toolkits/pages/engaginginsuccessionplanning.aspx

Turner, M. (n.d.). *Succession planning: Moving from discussion to execution* [PowerPoint slides]. Society for Human Resource Management. https://cr.shrm.org/sites/cr.shrm.org/files/Coleman%20Lew_Succession%20Planning.pdf

World Bank. (2020). *Unmasking the impact of COVID-19 on Businesses: Evidence from across the world.* https://openknowledge.worldbank.org/bitstream /handle/10986/34626/Unmasking-the-Impact-of-COVID-19-on-Businesses-Firm-Level-Evidence-from-Across-the-World.pdf?sequence=5&isAllowed=y

PART II

REMOTE WORKING CHALLENGES AND STRATEGIES

CHAPTER 12

HOW TO THRIVE WHILE WORKING FROM HOME

Terry Kibiloski

Whether you are telecommuting from home as an employee, running a home-based business, or freelancing from home, there are seven basic areas you need to get right to be successful:

- set yourself up for success in your home office environment;
- understand the basic technology you need;
- know how to keep you and your computer healthy;
- learn basic troubleshooting techniques;
- develop new skills and earn new certifications;
- control your own internet image; and
- understand how the internet has changed the hiring process.

SET YOURSELF UP FOR SUCCESS IN YOUR HOME OFFICE ENVIRONMENT

One of the first mistakes made by people working from home is not properly setting up their home office environment. This is not a new idea. Back in the 1880s, Frederick Winslow Taylor used time studies to improve

Back to a New Normal: In Search of Stability in an Era of Pandemic Disruption—Insight From Practitioners and Academics, pp. 163–182

the effectiveness of work, followed by Frank B. Gilbreth and Lillian M. Gilbreth who used time and motion studies to improve work efficiency. Using the same principles of these pioneers, it is amazing how small changes in your home office can help you become more effective and efficient, which can translate into using less time to perform tasks, and more income if you are a freelancer. For example, when I surveyed readers of *Computer Times* for home office failures and successes, I found that most failures came from lack of experience and planning. Let's look at a few examples below.

One of our readers shared that his and his wife's biggest failure was state-of-mind for both them and their two preteen children. Wishing to save on commute time and downtown office expenses, they moved their very successful consulting business to their home. They had their basement finished to basically look like the downtown office they just left. For the first few days, they walked down the stairs to their home office in whatever they happened to have on at the time, night clothes, casual clothes, etc. Within the first few weeks they realized that something was wrong. Their office hours seemed different in that they were quite lackadaisical toward their work, which was reflected in a decrease in income. Additionally, their children did not respect the fact that they were at work and thus the constant interruptions took time away from their consulting work. So, they began to dress for work, wearing the same business apparel they wore when their office was downtown. They also placed a sign on the door at the top of the steps that said "Do not disturb! Door does not open until 5 P.M." Soon, they saw their income return to normal and then increase. Their children learned that even though their parents moved their work location, their work hours remained the same. As they stated, even though they thought they had planned everything so perfectly, they did not initially understand the importance of state of mind.

Another reader shared that moving her office to her home was a disaster in that she was working twice as long to accomplish the same amount of work she used to do before telecommuting. In her case, her husband noticed the problem when she kept asking for things. For example, she would ask him to run out to the garage to get some paper for her printer, or ask him to find her a #2 pencil with an eraser, or ask him if he could get her some of the larger paper clips. He soon realized she had a totally unorganized home office which was leading to an unorganized life. She quickly did some research and reorganized her home office to where everything was in her immediate reach. She said she first did an inventory of everything she needed to efficiently do her job. She purchased all the needed supplies and equipment, including everything from a three-hole-punch to a multi-purpose printer that could make copies, scan documents to a flash drive, and send out faxes. She purchased a comfortable office chair, computer desk, footrest, small refrigerator, and coffee maker. She then set up her home office in the same efficient L-shape that she used to have in her downtown office. In front of her was a computer on a proper computer desk, with roll out keyboard shelf. Placed neatly on the computer desk was all the necessary peripheral equipment, everything within reach. To her left was a bookshelf with her multipurpose printer on top, a top shelf with her printer paper and ink cartridges, and all the small items she needed like pens, pencils, ruler, stapler, staple remover, sticky notes, scissors, etc. Her second shelf served as her inbox, with stacks of work in progress, while the bottom shelf became her outbox, with completed work and manuals. To the right of her computer desk was a small two-drawer filing cabinet and small fridge. On top of her filing cabinet was a small coffee maker. Once organized, she said that she completed her work in half the time, especially after adding headphones and having her computer play her favorite music.

A third reader shared that although he had his home office set up very efficiently, he had not prepared himself for everything he now needed to do without office and technical support. He first admitted that he had no idea how to send a package via the various national delivery services, or how to print postage on his printer to save going to the post office, or make a conference call, or send a fax through his computer, or clear a paper jam in his printer, or a host of other things that used to be done for him. Most importantly, he said that he did not know how to best stay in touch with his team, how to set up virtual meetings, or even how to log on and successfully interact in a virtual meeting. Sadly, he admitted that it took him too long to realize that his team was falling apart, needing more compassionate care, and mentoring, while working from home, and more specific instructions than ever before. Additionally, he sensed a lack of trust developing without the normal face-to-face human connections, so he began to send scanned personal notes to his team to regain that trust and was pleased to see others on the team do the same. Finally, he said he wished he could bill out the many hours he spent on YouTube learning how to do all the things he used to take for granted.

The above three examples should help you understand that thriving while working from home does not just magically happen. While you do save money on automotive expenses, clothes, and dry cleaning, and save time by not being in traffic each day, there are many other considerations you must make to accommodate your new work environment. With proper planning, though, working from home can be a very enjoyable and rewarding experience.

UNDERSTAND THE BASIC TECHNOLOGY YOU NEED

It is important to understand what basic technology you need and understand how that technology works. Depending upon what tasks you need to perform in your home office, you could possibly get by with a computer tablet and smartphone, or you may need a powerful desktop computer with multiple monitors, multipurpose printer, professional microphone, camera, LED studio lighting, and a drawing tablet for legible notes and signatures. Whatever technology you need, it is always useful to understand some basic things about computers in general.

Personal computers are not complicated. At first glance, the computer may appear to be a mysterious device filled with complex circuit cards, computer chips, and software. But if we break it down logically, the computer is not very complicated at all. Now, I am not talking about the genius behind the circuits and operating system that take a rocket scientist to understand, I'm talking about the basic operations of a computer.

When you look at a desktop or laptop computer, you see a keyboard, a monitor, and a case. The keyboard may look a little frightening at first, with all the specially marked keys, but let's follow its evolution. The first keyboards looked just like a typewriter, with only one extra button to send information to the computer. When the keyboard began to be used on personal computers, around the year 1982, users began to demand more keys. Accountants wanted a 10-key number pad (found at the far right of some keyboards), and game players wanted arrow buttons to direct their game movement (found embedded in the number pad, and repeated again between the number pad and the letter keys for the users who wanted quick access to both numbers and arrow keys). Users also began to demand special keys to do things like bold a word, *italicize a sentence*, and so on. Thus, the Control key was born (Ctrl on most keyboards). By pressing the Ctrl key at the same time you press another key, you can easily do things like bold (Ctrl + B), *italicize* (Ctrl + I), delete (Ctrl + X), copy (Ctrl + C), paste (Ctrl + V), and so on. These short cuts were great for touch typists who did not want to take their hands off the keyboard to use a mouse for the various tasks.

Soon, though, we ran out of key combinations and had to add an alternative control key, labeled the Alt key. When key combinations became a little confusing, users began to demand single keys to do specific functions, like bringing up "Help" information. Thus, the function keys were born (found at the top of the keyboard as F1, F2, etc.). Finally, we have the "Escape" (Esc) key (top left of keyboard) to help us escape from silly errors; the Delete and Insert keys (between the number pad and character keys) to delete and insert text; Home, End, Page Up/Down keys to quickly move through documents; and a few keys seldom used by most people, like Scroll Lock, Pause, and Print Screen (PrtScrn), the latter which will *not* print your screen in most situations but will take a snapshot of your screen so you can then paste a copy of your screen into a document, or into Paint, for more precise selection, copy, and paste.

The monitor is like your television. It has an on/off button, usually vertical/horizontal adjustments, contrast and brightness knobs, and image controls. It is rather simple to operate. Generally, the monitor control buttons are at the bottom right of the monitor, either facing front, or on the bottom of the monitor.

Finally, we have the computer case. The first thing you will notice is there are various sized slots on the sides (laptop) and back (laptop and desktop PC). Depending upon the model of your computer, you could also have a CD-ROM or a DVD drive, which can be used for playing CDs or DVDs, loading software, and creating backup DVDs to protect your data, picture, and video files. The various sized slots are used to plug in an external monitor, microphone, speakers, flash drives (also called memory sticks), and USB cords for charging your phone, cameras, and connecting other external devices.

Inside the computer are two important items, the hard drive, and the memory. The hard drive is used to record and save information on hard magnetic disks or on solid state drives (SSD). This is where your computer stores your application programs (word processor, spreadsheet, games, etc.) and your data files (documents, pictures, videos, etc.). The memory refers to several computer chips with millions/billions of tiny switches, used as the work area for the computer, which is also called the desktop.

Let's use a standard office desk for an analogy. The computer's hard disk is equivalent to the desk drawers, which can store hundreds of files. The computer's memory is equivalent to the top of the desk (desktop), where you can only work on a few files at a time. Both hard disks and memory are measured in bytes (equivalent to a character). A kilobyte (KB) is roughly a thousand characters; a megabyte (MB) is roughly a million characters; a gigabyte (GB) is roughly a billion characters. The more bytes available on your hard disk, the more files you can store. The more bytes available in memory (for the desktop), the more things you can work on at one time.

When buying a new computer, it is always a good rule to get as much memory and the largest hard drive that you can practically afford. You cannot buy too much memory or a hard drive too large. The more memory you have, the more things you can do at one time, and the faster your programs will run. The larger your hard drive, the more programs and information you can store. Just like you always seem to need a larger desk to hold all the things you are working on, and larger desk drawers to store all the things you want to store, you will always want more computer memory and hard drive space. You will never feel that you have too much memory to work on all the programs you want to use, or that you have enough hard drive space to store all the programs, pictures, videos, songs, and documents you want to store.

One of the largest hard drive hogs is your digital camera. Many digital camera owners leave their cameras on the default high resolution setting, and then only use their photos on the internet. High resolution images are only needed if you are going to print very large prints. Medium- or low-resolution photos are sufficient for internet viewing and up to 4×6 prints. The difference between high-resolution and low-resolution photos is incredible when it comes to how fast you fill up your camera's memory card, and your hard disk or flash drives for backups. So, it is a good idea to change your digital camera's default setting to medium- or low-resolution.

When purchasing a new laptop, tablet, or desktop PC, look for sales on those that use SSD memory rather than mechanical hard drives. SSD memory has no moving parts making it faster and more reliable. When powering up a laptop with SSD memory, it takes seconds rather than minutes.

KEEP YOU AND YOUR COMPUTER HEALTHY

Two common health risks for computer users are:

- computer vision syndrome; and
- carpal tunnel syndrome.

Computer Vision Syndrome

If you are a computer user and experience blurred vision, dry eyes, eye twitching, eye discomfort, headaches, neck and shoulder pain, and red eyes, you may have computer vision syndrome (Loh & Redd, 2008). A survey conducted by the Industrial Design Center, Indian Institute of Technology (Bali et al., 2007), shows that video display terminals, or computer work, is strenuous and leads to complex eye and vision problems. According to PubMed Central (PMC) at the U.S. National Institutes of Health's National Library of Medicine, nearly 60 million people worldwide suffer from computer vision syndrome. The American Optometric Association defines computer vision syndrome as a mix of eye and vision problems related to "near work," experienced during computer usage (Sheppard & Wolffsohn, 2018).

The Indian Institute of Technology study found that computer work is visually demanding, with the eye shifting and focusing between the screen, document, and keyboard 25,000 times a day. The eye must accommodate, converge, and adapt to these tasks under varying light of the internet, the report said. This task is equivalent to subjecting the eyes to 60 push-ups a minute.

Another study conducted by the Department of Human Factors Engineering, University of Occupational and Environmental Health, Japan, said that visual strain occurred after merely 60 minutes of internet tasks, which further resulted in lower productivity. While specially coated eyeglasses and anti-glare filters can reduce glare, there are other things you can do to reduce computer vision syndrome:

- Reduce the source of the glare. Adjust the lighting in your computer workspace by experimenting with turning on and off various lights, and repositioning those that can be moved. You might also try a variety of bulbs in your lights to achieve a softer lighting scheme. Close your window curtains or blinds to keep out the sun glare. Reposition your computer monitor. You could also buy an inexpensive flat screen monitor that plugs into the monitor port of your desktop or laptop personal computer.
- Invest in a large, high-resolution flat screen monitor. This will provide better visibility by accommodating larger font sizes and clearer images. This is an especially good option if you are constantly working with spreadsheets or extremely fine drawings or artwork. Your goal is to decrease eye strain and head and shoulder stress by allowing yourself to sit with good posture and view your monitor with its center point at eye level.
- Keep the monitor clean and free of dust, fingerprints, and smudges that can distort screen images. Never use water on your screen, or press into a flat screen monitor while cleaning, as this can damage the monitor's ability to present well-focused images. Invest in a box of inexpensive lint-free cleaning cloths made especially for flatscreen monitors and televisions.
- Rest and exercise your eyes at periodic intervals (every 20 minutes or so) by closing them for a few moments and then doing some refocusing exercises. The steps for refocusing exercises are as follows: Focus on an object close to your eyes (like a pencil or finger), focus on another object at arm's length, then focus on an object at a distance, repeating several times. When focusing on an object at a distance, without moving your head, go through the cycle of focusing to the top left, then top center, then top right (top being the

distant ceiling), continue the cycle of focusing to the center left, center, and center right (center being midway from ceiling to floor), then continue the cycle with bottom left, bottom center, and bottom right (bottom being near the floor). For example, focus on your finger as close to your face where you still have clear focus, then focus on a finger on your other hand at arm's length, then focus at a distance to the top left, then reverse to focus on your finger at arm's length, back to your finger close to your face, close your eyes for a moment, and begin this cycle again changing the distant focus to the top center, and so on. This will give your eye muscles a good overall workout, focusing at many distances and points, to compensate for your lengthy fixed focusing on your computer screen.

- Discuss computer vision syndrome with your ophthalmologist for further assistance and professional advice. It is important to have your eyes checked regularly to be sure that your blurred vision, dry eyes, eye twitching, eye discomfort, headaches, and red eyes, are not being caused by some physical eye disorder. It is especially important to have your eye pressure checked as high pressure can lead to a host of eye problems.

Another eye ailment mentioned by many computer users is red, irritated eyes. Studies have shown there is a decrease in blinking rate, plus wider opening of the eyes, when using a computer. This can result in fewer tears and greater tear evaporation, thus causing dry, irritated eyes. To relieve this problem, you may want to take frequent breaks, blink more, use mild eye drops, and maintain proper room humidity. A good temporary relief for tired, aching eyes, eye strain, burning and redness is the Similasan Computer Eye Relief sterile eye drops, which is formulated with natural active ingredients.

Carpal Tunnel Syndrome

Another major area of concern, many times associated with excessive computer use, is repetitive stress injury. The most common form of repetitive stress injury for computer users is called carpal tunnel syndrome. The carpal tunnel is a narrow passageway in the wrist through which nine tendons and the median nerve runs, which gives feeling to the hand. Many believe that with repetitive typing motion, the carpal tunnel tendons swell, and then compress and damage the sensitive median nerve, causing carpal tunnel syndrome. Keeping the wrists straight and using ergonomic aids may help prevent this condition.

Some doctors recommend expensive surgery to help fix the problem in severe cases. Unfortunately, some patients have found the surgery to be ineffective in solving the problem. Research suggests monitor position and posture, rather than repetitive motion, causes carpal tunnel syndrome. So, the question becomes "Are we treating symptoms and not the cause?"

POSITION OF HEAD, NOT WRIST ACTION, CAUSES CARPAL TUNNEL SYNDROME

According to some experts who specialize in computer workstation ergonomics, the improper placement of computer monitors causes the debilitating hand and arm injury that affects thousands of computer workers each year, commonly diagnosed as carpal tunnel syndrome (CTS). One researcher has gone as far to say constant strain on the neck from viewing improperly placed monitors 40 hours a week would cause CTS, even if the computer user never typed a single word.

Classic CTS symptoms are pain, numbness, and tingling in the hand, which can progress to a weakened grip and severe pain in the forearm or shoulder. CTS can worsen to the point where the nerves die. If this happens, the person's dysfunction of the hand or hands is irreversible, even with surgery.

What you may not realize is CTS also affects piano and violin players, hairdressers, knitters, telephone operators, cigar rollers, and grocery store clerks. Besides use of their hands in repetitive motions, these workers all have looking down in common, which can cause CTS, according to Julia Lacy, author of a book in its second printing, *How to Survive Your Computer Workstation* (Lacey et al., 1990). Another occupation affected by CTS is fish sorters who look down at fish on a conveyor belt and use a foot pedal rather than their hands to sort the fish.

Lacy says her conclusions come from surveys of several thousand full-time computer users over a 4-year period. Her theory is that looking down pitches the head forward, placing strain on the neck muscles, which in turn spasm. These spasms aggravate the nerve that emanates from beneath the seventh vertebra of the cervical spine from the C7/C8 nerve root area, which is connected to the median nerve. This eventually causes the symptoms associated with CTS (Lacey et al., 1990, p. 147).

"The head," says Lacy, "weighs as much as a bowling ball. Imagine the extra work neck muscles must do when the head moves off its natural pivot atop the shoulders," Lacy said. "When monitors are set too low," Lacy continues, "neck muscles must hold up a very heavy head, clamping down with a vicelike grip on the C5-TI area, home of nerves found along the arm. Eventually these exceedingly tense nerves spasm, shooting pain down the arm and into the wrist and hand, where ultimately their branches terminate."

Currently the medical profession still seems to focus on the wrist, with everything from splints to surgery. Before you have any intervention on your wrist, if you suffer from CTS symptoms, you may want to test Glick and Lacy's theory for yourself. A simple change in your monitor position and posture at your PC could save you a lot of pain and future expense. Personally, when I was experiencing CTS symptoms several years ago, adjusting monitor position and posture quickly fixed the problem.

PROTECT YOUR COMPUTER

The most common potential risks for your computer are human error, viruses, power surges, static, and lightning. The most effective way to protect your data against all these risks is to back up your data weekly, daily, hourly, or whenever you are at a point you cannot afford to lose it. We highly recommend using a high capacity Solid State Disk drive to continuously back up your entire hard disk. This allows you to quickly reconstruct your hard disk if your files are damaged or destroyed.

Unfortunately, backing up and restoring data is time consuming. So, the next best thing is to lower the odds of losing data. While human error is beyond the scope of this article, let's begin with helping you understand why "clean" power is important to your computer and how to protect your computer from power surges, brownouts, static, and lightning.

The computer is made up of thousands of tiny electrical switches. Each time you depress a key on the keyboard, a few of these switches are turned on to store the appropriate character in the computer's memory. The computer only has two choices for its switches, on or off, which are represented by the numbers 1 and 0. Think of a light switch. When you turn the switch to "on," the light comes on, represented by a 1 in a computer. When you turn the switch to "off," the light goes out, represented by a 0 in a computer.

The computer uses combinations of switches (1s and 0s) to store the various characters and numbers that we type through our keyboards. As an example, the letter "A" may be stored in eight switches in the following combination 11000001, and "C" may be stored as 11000011. The 1s represent a switch being on, and the 0s represent a switch being off.

Imagine a document of 2,000 characters you just typed into your word processor. Using our example, it would be using 16,000 switches in the computer's memory. Or, think of some of the larger programs that use a half million switches in your computer's memory to store their instructions. If even one of these switches is erroneously turned on by a power surge, or turned off by a momentary brownout, the information could be changed dramatically and give a spelling error in a document, or even "crash" the program.

Many times, this is what causes your keyboard to freeze up, or your program to stop working correctly. It could be caused by a microwave or coffeepot affecting your computer's power, or your coworker generating static electricity as they walk across the room and then touch you or your system, or even lightning that causes the power station to hiccup. Other static can come from a pet who walks across a carpet and then rubs against you while you're working at your computer or by you wearing clothes with material that creates static as you move in your chair. Computers, monitors, and printers are all affected by "dirty" electricity in the form of surges or brownouts, a sudden loss of electricity, or static.

A few things you can do to help prevent these conditions are:

- **Plug your computer, and all components, into a surge suppressor.** You might also think about a whole house surge suppressor that is installed at your electricity panel. For a couple hundred dollars, you can have all the plugs in your house surge protected.
- **Do not run power hogs on the same circuit as your computer,** like coffeepots, microwaves, space heaters, and window air conditioners.
- **Consider buying a quality uninterruptible power supply (UPS).** Then, if your main power goes out, your UPS will give you enough time (15 minutes to an hour depending on the model) to safely save your working files. Many UPS products come with software that can detect a power outage and safely save your files, and safely power down your computer, even if you are not home.
- **Use a simple room humidifier** to decrease the amount of static electricity in the immediate area of your computer.
- **Back up your files often** to provide easy recovery in case the above precautions do not provide enough protection.

BASIC TROUBLESHOOTING TECHNIQUES

In addition to the various ways we just discussed about protecting your computer, you should learn some basic troubleshooting techniques to keep your technology running when you most need it. Many of the costly repairs and support service failures that computer users require each year can easily be prevented, or cured, by the computer users themselves. The old saying, "An ounce of prevention is worth a pound of cure," can be applied to computers in the words "*a little disaster prevention is worth a lot of disaster recovery.*" In fact, a little disaster prevention may be required to even begin disaster recovery. A couple of examples follow *(the names are omitted to protect the victims).*

A home business that relied heavily on customer contacts to maintain a steady cash flow suffered a fire that destroyed computers, files, and all magnetic media. Although they did a backup of their entire system each night, they did not maintain any backup tapes or disks off site. There was virtually no way to recover from this disaster and continue to stay in business. It is so important to have multiple backups of your files, in multiple locations. In addition to the fire scenario, sometimes disaster can strike when the backup media cannot be used by the computer due to a faulty flash drive, scratched DVD, or a failed backup drive. Be creative with your off-site backup locations. Some that have been used are a safe deposit box, bowling alley locker, spare tire well of vehicle, and grandparents' house, the latter providing a nice daily visit with the grans. If you are comfortable having strangers in charge of backing up your data, consider using internet "cloud" backup plans.

Another example is a home-based business, that relied heavily on internet connections, and suffered a loss of online sales for two weeks, severely affecting their cash flow, which nearly caused bankruptcy. In this situation, a car accident destroyed a major piece of routing equipment for the internet provider that required days to replace. It is important to understand that when you are at the mercy of an outside provider, you must have an automatic backup. In this case, the home-based business should have had two internet service providers, which is a relatively small extra cost to pay for dependable internet support.

While the above two examples were disaster prevention techniques, how do you cure technology problems that slow or prevent you from using your computer? The best solution, in many situations, is to follow a simple troubleshooting plan. Here are a few steps to follow.

- **Identify the problem as specifically as possible.** Then, open Google and search for the *key words* of your problem. If your computer is not operational, use your smartphone for the search. Read several articles and watch several videos to find a consensus to solving your problem. Then, follow the instructions to see if they will solve your problem.
- ***Do not* feel compelled to find the specific cause** of a one-time problem IF you can quickly recover by simply restarting your computer. Many hours can be wasted by playing detective and trying to pinpoint the exact cause of a fatal system error or system lockup.

Often these errors are caused by an unidentifiable cause like a power flux or static. Unless the same problem continues to occur, simply restart your computer, and get on with your computer tasks. If a system restart does not work, power the system off, wait ten seconds for all switches to return to zero and all moving parts to stop, then power the system on. This will usually fix 99% of the problems since powering on has the operating system do multiple system checks, with automatic reinstalls of anything that is not working correctly.

- **If your problem is still not resolved, power your system off completely.** If you are using a laptop computer, simply selecting the Shut Down feature, or pressing the Power button on your laptop, will not completely shut down your computer. Laptop computers run on batteries so even if you power it down, the battery is still providing power to the laptop. For a complete shutdown, you need to unplug the power cord and remove the battery for a few seconds. Then, place the battery back in place, and plug in the power cord.
- **After a *complete* power off, power on your computer so it can complete a cold boot.** A cold boot, also called a hard boot, resets all the switches to zero, clearing out random-access memory, which contains counters, pointers, and internal data created by the operating system and programs. In effect, everything is started from scratch. A cold boot begins with a small set of instructions in the BIOS, or UEFI in newer systems, which are stored in read-only memory, that tests the hardware, loads in key configuration data, and then finds, loads, and starts the operating system. So, if your initial problem had anything to do with a power surge, static, or any other situation that caused errors in the operating system or programs that you were running, a cold boot should resolve your issue.
- **Consider buying a new computer before repairing your old one**. Do not spend many dollars in lost time to save a few dimes in hardware or software. Sometimes the easiest cure is to replace the hardware, reload working copies of your programs and files from your best backup, and get on with it. If it does make good financial sense to repair the hardware, consider renting a system in the interim. Generally, though, it makes more sense to buy new equipment. With the ever-decreasing price, and increasing power, of today's computers, monitors, and printers, a small investment in new equipment can return large dividends in productivity.

DEVELOP NEW SKILLS AND EARN NEW CERTIFICATIONS

If you read the earlier sections of this chapter, you may have already developed some new skills in successfully setting up a home office, knowing how a computer works, keeping yourself and your computer safe, and troubleshooting computer problems. So, how do you translate these skills, and others you might have, into recognized certifications that can help you advance in your current organization, secure a better job in another organization, or increase your credibility as a home business owner or a freelancer? In most cases, it is easier than you might think.

If you are working from home, there is a good chance you are already proficient with one or more Microsoft Office programs. If you feel that you are fairly proficient in using these programs, the first place to look for certifications for which you might already qualify is https://docs.microsoft.com/en-us/learn/certifications/browse/. At this website, you will find Microsoft Office Specialist certifications for Microsoft Word, Excel, PowerPoint, Access, Outlook, and OneNote, to name a few. Plus, there are multiple certifications for Microsoft 365 for everything from fundamentals to teams administrator associate. Additionally, you will find several certifications for Microsoft Dynamics, Azure, Windows, and more. In short, you will find multiple pages of available certifications, with a filter option to help you find the best certifications for you.

In addition to Microsoft certifications, there are many other industry certifications that you can readily obtain. Some of the more popular are certifications for computer hardware, other computer software products, first aid, human resources, languages, marketing, programming, project management, and notary public. A couple of internet searches for certifications in your industry will undoubtedly reveal many more.

While some certifications require a set time of experience, many simply require you to pass an online exam. For each certification, you will find multiple sources for study guides and online training. Before spending any money on methods to help prepare you for a certification exam, visit the website of the certifying company (i.e., Microsoft) or industry organization (i.e., Red Cross) to find free study guides and a list of tasks you need to know to pass the exam.

If you are already working from home, especially if you have the type of job that requires you to wait at your computer for things like virtual team meetings, replies from customers, and so on, seriously consider filling in that wait time with the pursuit of multiple certifications. Also, consider completing Skillsoft courses and achieving Skillsoft certifications. Many companies use Skillsoft courses to train their employees in a host of skills related to business, compliance, productivity, collaboration, and technology. If you have been trained by your company using a Skillsoft course, you may find that you already have access to many other Skillsoft courses. Check with your Human Resources department.

Part of thriving while working from home is using time management to work on a variety of ways to increase your skills, obtain certifications, and increase your overall value to your current employer, future employer, customers, and clients. Even if you have no interest in certifications, at least watch a few YouTube videos each day that cover a variety of new information for your industry and career field. There are many very professional YouTube videos that can teach you a host of new skills and provide new knowledge in a series of 5-minute videos.

CONTROL YOUR OWN INTERNET IMAGE

Let's begin this section with a question. Are you happy with the professional image that you portray to the world each day? If you are interested in thriving while working at home, it is important to understand that LIFE is an interview, continuously creating the professional image that you portray to the world. The fact is, we are observed by many people each day, in a variety of settings, each assessing us through our body language, our actions, our behavior, our dress, and a variety of other observable qualities. This continuous professional image creation rapidly takes place in our digital life on the internet, especially as we work from home and spend countless more hours on the internet.

It might be a good time to review your digital footprint. I suggest you do an internet search for YOU! Type in various names you have used over the years, both professionally and casually, and your city of residence. Are you proud of what appears? Would you be okay with your digital life on the front page of your local newspaper? It is important to understand that everything you do on the internet is stored and recoverable by creditors, investigative reporters, lawyers, bankers, and human resource professionals who are screening you for potential employment. That includes every e-mail, tweet, text, post, search, like, dislike, and so on. Are you happy with the image that your digital footprint portrays?

It is important to understand that when Shakespeare compared the world to a stage, and stated that we were actors upon that stage, he was not referring to a single role. How many roles have you played today? I suggest that it is many more than you might think. When I ask a classroom of students to give me all the roles that they each play on any given day, the count gets up to 30 or more: parent, wife, mother, student, driver, shopper, patient, and so on. Each role tends to have an unspoken set of rules and results in outward displays of a different set of behaviors, values, and morals. Do you behave the same way in church as you do at a party? Do you behave the same way on the internet as you do in a professional setting?

It is important to have your collective behavior, in all settings, reflect the person you want the world to see. With the instant videos, texts, tweets, e-mails, and social media posts that are retrievable to anyone via the internet, we have lost a great deal of privacy in our daily lives. It is amazing how many job candidates are dismissed because of behaviors far removed from their professional lives, including their behaviors in a bar, at a party, on the internet, and in traffic. While we do play a variety of roles each day, it is important that we learn to show a consistent set of behaviors, values, and morals across all of them

I suggest you begin to consciously think about every search, like, dislike, post, survey, opinion, and so many other digital footprint breadcrumbs you are leaving each day on the internet. This includes the websites you visit, the videos you view, and the products and services you purchase. To have a better understanding of how much information is collected about you each day via the internet, I suggest you watch the trailer of the Netflix (2019) documentary titled *The Great Hack*. The trailer, and the full documentary, will both educate you and shock you on how virtually everything you do on the internet is tracked by analytic companies for the purpose of creating a deeply personal profile of you that they can sell for big money. This is not new. Information has been more valuable than gold, oil, or any other precious commodity for a long time.

So, what do you do if you have a less than professional image on the internet? I suggest you begin to actively control your digital image. Begin by creating a very professional LinkedIn profile, taking the time to populate every possible aspect of your profile, from professional achievements to education to skills. Be sure to list every school you ever attended, and every social and professional group to which you belonged, including early groups like boy scouts, girl scouts, science club, and so on. LinkedIn is all about links. The more information you have in your profile, the more people you will be able to link to who share common experiences with you. The general rule is the more links the better. If you want instant access to many people, request that I link with you on LinkedIn (Dr. Terry Kibiloski). Then, you will have access to all my links. Additionally, join all the professional groups on LinkedIn that correspond to your job, career, and industry. This will link you to professionals to whom you can relate. Not only will this provide more contacts, it will also provide a source of helpful opinions and information from professionals in your industry.

The next thing you can do to control your own internet image is to create a personal professional website using a free website creation platform like wix.com. If you can use Microsoft Word, you can create a website. Through your own professional website, you can share professional photos, videos, and other things you have created or accomplished, like PowerPoint presentations, research papers, and so on. You will be able to show people not only who you are but what you can do. In short, you are making it easy for people to see your professional self in the manner you wish to be observed. As you create your LinkedIn profile, and your professional website, be sure to watch several YouTube videos that will show you how to do so in the best way possible.

HOW THE INTERNET HAS CHANGED THE HIRING PROCESS

If you have not recently applied for a job, created a resume, or been interviewed, be aware that the hiring process has been dramatically changed by the internet. This is true whether you are seeking a new job, applying for a new position in your current company, being considered for a promotion, or being interviewed as a freelancer. In a matter of moments, after you submit a job application on the internet, a computer can determine whether you will be rejected or not. Yes, you will receive an acknowledgment of your application being received, but the fate of your application may be determined by the key words you used in your application and resume rather than by your actual skills, experience, and education. With so many job applications being submitted for advertised jobs, the first task of the hiring manager is to cut down the hundreds, or possibly thousands, of applications to a manageable few. This requires artificially intelligent software using key word searches and word matches.

So, what can you do to help your application and resume pass the computer key word search test? It all begins with the job description advertised on the internet. If you are logged into one of the many online recruiting sites, be sure to print out the job description in its entirety, including the responsibilities and tasks for the position being offered, plus the desired skills and experience for the job candidate. Then, log on to the website of the specific company that is advertising the job opening. For example, even though you may have found the job on a website like ziprecruiter.com, if it is a job with UPS, go directly to the UPS corporate website, scroll down, and click on *Careers*. When the *Careers* webpage opens, put in the search criteria for the advertised job. When you find that job, print out the job description in its entirety, like you did at the online recruiting site. Then, compare the two job description printouts.

Often, the corporate *Careers* website will have more detailed and up-to-date information on the advertised job. The first thing to look for is if the job is still open. Even though it shows up on an online recruiting site, if the corporate site shows it as no longer available, it is a waste of time to apply via the online recruiting site. The next thing to look for are any differences between the two job descriptions. Generally, the corporate site will have the most detailed job description. Using a colored highlighter, highlight each of the key words, in both of your printed job descriptions, that identify the specific requirements, skills, and experience for the job. Examples of key words would be *problem solver*, *programmer*, *Gofast* (fictitious programming language for this article), *Microsoft Word*, and so on.

Each of the highlight key words *must* be on your job application and in your resume. You want to have a direct match for every key word that the artificially intelligent software uses to determine if an application is accepted or not. Also, be sure to use the exact spellings. If the job description states that you must be proficient in *Microsoft Word*, do not simply put *MS Word*, or just *Word* in your application and resume. Also, if the job description list multiple *Microsoft* products like Word, Excel, PowerPoint, and Access, and you happen to be a Certified Microsoft Office Specialist, do not just list these four words on your application and resume. While a human being might know that a Certified Microsoft Office Specialist would be proficient in the four Microsoft applications mentioned, an artificially intelligent software package might only be programmed for direct word matches. So, in this case, I suggest you list both, your Microsoft certification, for the human resource personnel who may actually read your application and resume if it is accepted by the software, and the key words for the software to be sure your application is accepted. So, your bulleted item on your resume might be—Certified Microsoft Office Specialist (Microsoft Word, Excel, PowerPoint, Access, etc.). This way you are covered for both the software and the human reviewer.

The same would be true in your narrative description of your skills. If the job description says *problem solver*, be sure to use that phrase. So, instead of saying "I love to solve problems," use the term *problem solver* in a list of your strong points. In our example above, this would hold true for the term *programmer* and *Gofast*. What do you do, though, if you never even heard of the Gofast programming language. Quickly go to YouTube and search for *Gofast*. If it is a relatively new programming language, or simply one you have not yet encountered, there will certainly be instructive videos available for you to watch. You might also do a Google search for *Gofast videos*. Once you watch a few videos about Gofast, you can honestly include a bullet on your resume that states—*Currently learning Gofast*. In this way, you are not being deceitful, and you have the keyword *Gofast* on your resume for a keyword software match.

Let's move forward in your job search process. If your application and resume get past the artificially intelligent software keyword search process, you might be automatically set up by the same software to do an internet video interview. You will still be working directly with a computer at this point. Generally, you will be given a link to the video interview platform and directed to complete the interview by a certain date. While a computer will be recording the video interview, be assured that if you meet the selection criteria in the video interview a human being will eventually critique your video interview for future selection, for a live phone interview, or maybe even a person-to-person interview. So, what do you need to know about a video interview?

When you click the link for the video interview, you will generally be linked to a video interview website that will first check your computer to be sure your camera and microphone are working. If there is a problem, you may be given tips on what to do on your computer to get them both working. Once your camera and microphone get the "green light" you will be provided some practice questions so you can become familiar with how the questions are asked, and where to look on the screen for the countdown before the recording starts (3, 2, 1, ...) and where to see the clock recording the time of your answer. This is important because if you are given 2 minutes as the maximum time to reply, the recording will quit at exactly 2 minutes. Generally, you can do as many practice sessions as needed. A typical question will be presented as a video on your screen showing a person describing a scenario and then asking you a question, sometimes a multi-part question. For example, the person on the video might say "This job requires you to be a problem solver since there are so many different things that can occur from day to day. Describe a time when you needed to be a problem solver to get the job done."

In your recorded answers, be sure you use the STAR technique (Situation, Task, Action, Result). Briefly describe the *Situation* (i.e., I once had an angry customer approach me who wanted to return a product for a cash refund of $100 even though it was past our usual 30-day return policy), then describe your *Task* (i.e., I knew I needed to first calm down the customer and then do my best to make her happy), then your *Action* (i.e., So, I told her that while company policy would not allow me to do a cash return, I could give her an in-store credit for $100, and could also give her 50% off on her next purchase, to allow her to buy an even better product for her money), and finally describe the *Result* (i.e., Not only did I make the customer happy, she continued to shop at our store and always asked for me to help her with her purchases.) While giving your answer, be sure you keep tabs on the 2-minute clock, so you don't go past the time and have your recorded answer get cut off.

Understand that a video interview requires some "stage" preparation. Be sure the background behind you is staged to look professional. A plain background is always good, but you could also have a background that suits the job for which you are applying. For example, if you have a nice, professional office shown as your background, that could show that you are organized. Be very cautious that you eliminate anything in the background that could be viewed negatively. Finally, look your professional best, including your hair, makeup, nails, clothes, eyeglasses, etc. Most importantly, when you are recording your answers look directly at the camera with lots of positive smiles and demonstrate confidence in your answers. Not only do you want to look professional, but you also want to look friendly so the person reviewing your video sees someone with whom they would like to work. From a technical point of view, be sure you have adequate lighting that is positioned properly. You will find many YouTube videos that will show you the best positioning for 3-point LED lighting to best illuminate your face.

THRIVING WHILE WORKING FROM HOME SUMMARY

If you read this entire chapter, you now know how to thrive while telecommuting, running a home-based business, or freelancing from home. Just stay focused on the seven key areas below and you will thrive beyond your wildest dreams.

- set yourself up for success in your home office environment;
- understand the basic technology you need;
- know how to keep you and your computer healthy;
- learn basic troubleshooting techniques;
- develop new skills and earn new certifications;
- control your own internet image; and
- understand how the internet has changed the hiring process.

REFERENCES

Bali, J., Navin, N., & Thakur, B. R. (2007). Computer vision syndrome: A study of the knowledge, attitudes and practices in Indian ophthalmologists. *Indian Journal of Ophthalmology, 55*(4), 289–294. https://doi.org/10.4103/0301-4738.33042

Lacey, J. S., Dickson, T., & Levinson, H. A. (1990). *How to survive your computer workstation: 15 Easy steps to workstation comfort.* CRT Services.

Loh, K., & Redd, S. (2008). Understanding and preventing computer vision syndrome. Malaysian family physician: *The Academy of Family Physicians Journal of Malaysia, 3*(3), 128–130.

Netflix. (2019). *The great hack.* [Documentary picture]. United States: Netflix. https://www.netflix.com/title/80117542

Sheppard, A. L., & Wolffsohn, J. S. (2018). Digital eye strain: prevalence, measurement, and amelioration. *BMJ Open Ophthalmology, 3*(1), e000146. https://doi.org/10.1136/bmjophth-2018-000146

CHAPTER 13

A WHOLE NEW BALL GAME

Motivating and Managing a Remote Workforce

Helen MacLennan

The COVID-19 pandemic completely changed the way many of us live and work. Fear of viral spread guidelines around social distancing eliminated our ability to work together in the same spaces and the only option for many businesses was to move business operations online. Entire industries scrambled to do what was necessary to prepare their workforces to work from home. Managing these remote employees brought a host of new issues including employment law changes, increased security concerns, and social isolation that made motivating and managing employees a new challenge—one for which management may have been unprepared.

Early in the transition, employees realized they were not going to be required to be in the office every day and many looked forward to a greater sense of freedom and autonomy along with the opportunity to spend more time with their families. Childcare and traffic were no longer going to be a struggle; and work clothes were going to become much more comfortable. However, what they may not have realized was that after more than a year of working remotely, they would likely be strug-

Back to a New Normal: In Search of Stability in an Era of Pandemic Disruption—Insight From Practitioners and Academics, pp. 183–200

gling with feelings of isolation and a lack of motivation (Burroughs, 2020; Chewka, 2018; Grenny & Maxfield, 2017; Place, 2021). Their managers are struggling too.

When preparing to transition workforces to remote locations, organizations focused on training management and workforces on new technology, procedures, and processes. Many would learn about the benefits and nuances of remote communications using video conferencing software such as Zoom, Microsoft Teams, GoToMeeting and Skype. So—one year later, managers probably have a firm grasp on the technical aspects of their jobs, but may be struggling with work-life balance, employee satisfaction and productivity, employee communication, and social isolation. The best managers have learned that motivating and managing a remote workforce requires a unique approach and a different set of managerial skills (Parker et al., 2020). Managing employees through the pandemic became a whole new ball game.

Remote employees are likely to be struggling with a host of things that can negatively influence overall motivation and productivity. Some of their primary struggles include:

- Social isolation (Bucurean, 2020; Grenny & Maxfield, 2017; Lowy, n.d.; Nedelcu, 2020);
- Work-life balance (Kurowska, 2018; Parker et al., 2020; Rocco, 2020; van der Lippe & Lippenyi, 2018);
- Loss of face to face communication (Lowy, 2020);
- Unnecessary meetings (Lowy, 2020);
- Childcare issues (Lobell & Lobell, 2020; Mercado, 2020);
- Lack of organization (Bucurean, 2020; Nedelcu, 2020);
- Erosion of work/home boundaries (Bucurean, 2020; Koslowski et al., 2019; Kurowska, 2018; Nedelcu, 2020);
- Inadequate work environment (Koslowski et al., 2019);
- Emotional exhaustion (Huang & Chang, 2020; Rocco, 2020);
- Distractions at home (Reuschke et al., 2021); and
- Job insecurity (Chapman et al., 2020; Jung et al., 2021).

The issues surrounding remote work appear to center around these 4 broad categories. The following sections will include an overview of how work has changed for those working remotely; the issues with which they struggle and how those issues might negatively impact motivation and productivity. I will also offer management tips for helping the reader to better connect, motivate and manage your remote workforce, while pro-

Figure 13.1

Remote Work Issues

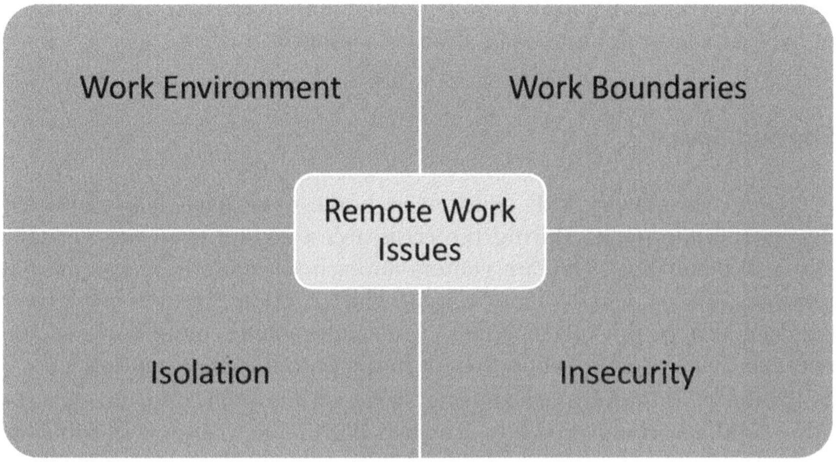

tecting your organization. Here is where you can begin developing your remote managerial skills.

WORK ENVIRONMENT

When employees were asked to begin working from home in response to the pandemic, many were unprepared and unequipped. You may have provided them with a company-owned computer, but your remote employees may lack an adequate work environment in their home. Many do not have a desk or dedicated workspace in their homes, leaving them to struggle with issues of organization, security, and comfort.

Prior to the move to remote work, your employees probably had adequate workspaces—a desk, cubicle, or office. However, now almost 75% of 1,000 American remote workers surveyed indicated that they had worked from their bed during the pandemic (Lufkin, 2021). For some, it may be their only option. Unfortunately, working from a bed for an extended period, can result in physical health issues, including sleep problems, such as insomnia or circadian rhythm disorder. That lack of sleep is negatively impacting employee productivity (Lufkin, 2021).

While technology has afforded us the ability to work apart from one another, you should consider that for your employees—all things may not be equal. Remote workers may be sharing their space with others in the home who are working remotely and with children, who are learning remotely. Unless your organization has provided employees with personal computers, they may also have the need to share equipment with others in the household. In addition, your remote employees may lack access to, or be able to afford, high-speed internet connections.

Sharing Space

Remote employees with children at home were particularly affected during the pandemic. During the crisis access to childcare was virtually eliminated for most. Daycare centers and schools closed, or operated at reduced capacity, leaving many parents with no choice than to bring their children into the workplace. Failure to accommodate remote working parents can cause resentment and result in the potential for litigation.

If remote employees are sharing space with young children, pets, or other adults working remotely, which is highly likely, they will probably have increased sound, interruptions, and work distractions during the workday. All of which can negatively influence job performance and satisfaction (Johanson, 2021) and contribute to work burnout (Westfall, 2020). Keep in mind that excessive noise and inadequate workspaces are highlighted in videoconference meetings. Consider that employees on camera may feel anxious about the background noise or embarrassed about sharing their surroundings with coworkers and management.

Management Tips

You certainly cannot be expected to provide a dedicated workspace for your employees who work from home. However, there are some things you can do to help alleviate the negative impacts of inadequate workspaces.

- Let your employees know that you understand that background noise can often not be helped.
- In virtual meetings, allow employees to have their cameras off, if necessary.
- Try not to single out employees who may have small children at home or other excessive background noise. Instead, ask and ask that all employees keep their microphones off when not speaking.
- Eliminate unnecessary videoconference meetings. Consider that these may add additional stress and anxiety for your employees.

- Be flexible. If possible, provide daily or weekly assignments and appropriate deadlines. Allow the employee to work flexible hours.
- Engage in ongoing dialogue with your team. It may be the only way to ensure your employees have everything they need to be productive.
- If possible, allow employees to expense the cost of internet or equipment they need to be productive.

Remote management skills required: empathy, flexibility, connection.

Security

Sharing workspace also presents heightened issues surrounding privacy and security. Trade secrets, proprietary and financial information, and cyber-security become more difficult to control in unsecured remote environments. Employees may save proprietary or financial information to personal devices, print secured documents at home, send company information to personal email addresses, and utilize unsecured personal networks and computer devices (Csercevits, 2021).

Intellectual property attorney, Thomas McNulty indicated that protecting trade secrets where employees work remotely has at least three separate and distinct issues: security and integrity of data networks and communications systems; security of remote workplaces; the ability to retrieve sensitive data and prevention of its misappropriation when employment ends (Lando, 2020). All of these put your organization at an increased risk of security breaches.

The pandemic has certainly caused a significant increase in the use of videoconferencing, which presents another security issue. The *National Law Review* (2021) indicated that at least one court declined to extend trade secret protection to proprietary information discussed during virtual meetings based on the businesses' lack of action to take reasonable steps to protect the information. When employees are working remotely, securing documents and information takes more stringent measures.

Management Tips

Begin with a security audit, which should include a review of all existing policies and procedures. Work to revise policies, as necessary to address issues specific to remote work in order to help increase security and protection of data. Lando (2020) suggests implementing the following:

- Develop or revise existing employment agreements to include confidentiality and non-disclosure agreements.
- Provide company-owned computers with security software to all employees.
- Restrict access to confidential and proprietary data.
- Require all work be completed on company issued computers.
- Require employees to connect to the organization through an encrypted network with specific password requirements.
- Take steps to ensure the security of virtual meetings.
- Provide training on best practices to secure data.

Remote management skills required: knowledge, communication.

Employment Law

Your remote employees may be living in other states. Consequently, different employment and tax laws may apply. For instance, income tax requirements may vary from state to state as well as minimum wage and overtime pay laws. In addition, new employment legislation exists in response to the pandemic.

The Families First Coronavirus Response Act provides for 12 weeks of emergency family and medical leave to be used to care for the employees' child(ren) because their school or daycare was closed or unavailable due to the pandemic. Organizations that violate the law by denying leave to qualifying employees could find themselves in private litigation or being sued by the U.S. Department of Labor (Lobell, 2020).

Unless your nonexempt employees are excluded from the Fair Labor Standards Act, you will need to implement procedures to track working hours and ensure that they are paid 1.5 times their regular rate of pay for any time worked over 40 hours in a work week. prevent violations of overtime laws. Even if your employees work without being asked, you may have to pay them overtime if they do (Garrison, 2021).

Regardless of where your employees are physically located, laws regarding discrimination, such as the Americans with Disabilities Act, Title VII of the Civil Rights Act, and the Equal Pay Act, still apply (Garrison, 2021). For instance, if a disabled employee is required to work from home, you will be required to provide reasonable accommodations that will allow them to perform their job remotely.

When it comes to on-the-job injuries, the remote location can be considered to be an extension of the workplace. A remote employee will generally be entitled to workers' compensation if the worker was injured performing work-related activities (Garrison, 2021). Consequently, if your employee is injured while at work in their home, you may be subject to the same liability as if it happened in the workplace.

During the pandemic, as many as 25 states have also enacted new regulations regarding paid sick time, workers' compensation, vacation, minimum wage and employee scheduling. It is critical that you know where your employees are working and for how long to help ensure compliance with new and existing employment regulations. Management should consider the following tips:

- Familiarize yourself with new employment laws.
- Set clear work hours.
- Set policies against working off the clock and unapproved overtime.
- Set clear guidelines for employee job duties.
- Require employees to track and report time worked.

Remote management skills required: knowledge, communication.

WORK BOUNDARIES

One of the biggest changes your workforce has likely experienced is that they are working in their home environment and technology allows them to be continually connected to work. Employees who work physically on site typically enjoy a clear demarcation of work time and personal time. Unfortunately, in the current environment, that is not the case for most of the workforce. In a recent study, more than 80% of employees indicated that said they had more stress and anxiety this year as work issues spilled over into personal life due to a lack of boundaries (Johanson, 2021). Boundaries refer to the clear separation of work and life.

Frequent interruptions and distractions occur when working from home, particularly if there are children, pets, or other individuals present. Meal preparation, household chores, children's homework, and pet care become interwoven into the workday. Consequently, the lines between work and home time have become blurred. Assignments may not get completed during traditional work hours and employees may find themselves working non-traditional hours in order to complete their assignments.

As work and life can easily meld when working remotely, your employees are likely to be struggling with work-life balance. Many remote employees indicate receiving texts and emails early morning and late at night, making it necessary to constantly check emails and phones. A recent report indicates that one of the biggest issues faced by remote employees is unplugging after work (Buffer, 2021). Videoconferencing can also break down boundaries between professional and personal life. Compare it to having your work team into your home several times a week—or per day. Your employees may be uncomfortable sharing their surroundings or suffer feelings of embarrassment when children, roommates or family members unexpectedly join their virtual meetings. Employees can also feel vulnerable to explicit and implicit comparisons of their personal workspaces (Johanson, 2021).

Management Tips

Just because technology has enabled you to reach your employees at all times of the day *does not mean you should*. Consider which meetings can be turned into emails, reducing the infringement on their time and productivity. Be understanding and flexible. With the additional home and family responsibilities your employees may have during the workday, it can be unrealistic to expect them to be continually at their computers or to immediately respond to phone calls or emails. Also, with the lines between work and home blurred, resist the urge to call or send emails well past working hours.

- Set clear and realistic expectations around work deadlines.
- Expect and encourage frequent work breaks.
- Be flexible—allowing work to be completed on their schedule, when possible.
- Respect work hours and resist the urge to meet, text or email after hours.
- Set boundaries for yourself and communicate them to others.
- Turn unnecessary meetings into emails.

Remote management skills required: communication, flexibility.

ISOLATION

The pandemic has forced many to work from home for much longer than they had originally anticipated. The combination of being physically separated from coworkers, experiencing reduced access to information and materials, and a lack of recognition for their individual contributions can make employees lose a real connection to their work.

Add to that the closure of local restaurants, bars, movie theaters, and other small businesses and it becomes understandable that remote employees report their largest concern as feelings of loneliness and social isolation (Hickman, 2019; Modi, 2019; Moss, 2020).

Because workplaces can be a primary source of friends and acquaintances and these social connections are crucial to psychological health, remote workers may be suffering. In fact, Nicholas Bloom, a researcher on remote working, indicated that the answer to why half of remote workers indicated a desire to return to the workplace was social company. Marital status, living arrangements, and a lack of social networks can make some remote employees more susceptible to loneliness due to social isolation. He added that "I fear an extended period of working from home will not only kill office productivity but is building a mental health crisis" (cited in Gorlick, 2020).

Not only is the mental health of your remote employees at risk when working remotely, loneliness and social isolation can cause physical health problems as well. Both have been found to be linked to sleep problems (Benson et al., 2021; McLay et al., 2021), which will certainly negatively influence employee productivity. The Centers for Disease Control and Prevention indicate that long-term isolation can not only result in increased rates of anxiety and depression, but has negative health effects that rival those of smoking and obesity (2020a, 2020b).

Communication

Communication and connecting with employees become critical when they are working remotely. Technology has made it easy to connect virtually with remote workers, however, some managers have taken advantage of that. Excessively frequent or unproductive meetings take away valuable work time from your employees, causing unnecessary stress and anxiety. In a recent discussion with remote employees, they indicated they used the time in virtual conferences to shop online, read, answer emails, or handle household chores.

Remote employees are also likely to experience feelings of disconnection from their workplace. In a downward spiral, lower affiliation with work results in a tendency for employees to withdraw and reduce their commitment to the organization, resulting in a decrease in job performance (Ozcelik & Barsade, 2018). Getting information to your remote employees is important. However, they can also struggle with information overload, particularly if news and information is coming from a combination of emails, virtual bulletin boards, and social media outlets. They may struggle with the constant fear of missing something if information is coming from all directions.

As your remote employees work separately and more autonomously, information silos can often occur—when information isn't shared between individuals or departments. Employees who lack the information they need to perform their jobs effectively, they may experience frustration or make uninformed decisions that can negatively impact the entire organization. Separation of the workforce makes it more difficult for your employees to stay aware of what everyone else is doing.

Workplace Culture

Working remotely in separate physical spaces and being isolated from co-workers has served to change many workplace cultures. While the daily tasks may have remain unchanged, no longer are your employees exposed to the daily face to face interactions or the rituals shared within the office. The Strategic Human Resources Management organization indicates that "Organizations should be concerned about watering down their culture by relying solely on asynchronous communication" and suggest that organizations who fail to undertake the work necessary to maintain their culture or purposefully steer it in a new direction will struggle with unpredictable results (Hinds & Elliott, 2021).

Management Tips

Gallup recommends five distinct types of conversations that drive performance. You should be having these conversations with your employees to make them feel more connected and engaged. They include: a quick-connect; check-in; developmental coaching; progress review; and role/relationship development (Hickman, 2019). Used together, they can provide an opportunity for you to better understand and connect with your remote employees, making them feel more connected to the organization.

- Use the five types of conversations.
- Create opportunities for remote socialization.
- Schedule small in-person gatherings, if possible.
- Be available and allow for open communication.
- Avoid unnecessary meetings.

- Choose a dedicated method for disseminating information.
- Elicit employee opinions.
- Recognize individual employee contributions.

Remote management skills required: communication, connection.

INSECURITY

Working remotely, disconnected from coworkers, can lead to feelings of insecurity. In fact, during the pandemic, your remote employees are likely dealing with a host of insecurities surrounding their futures, jobs, health, access to food and supplies, and the overall economy. Unless your employees are cut off from the outside world, they will be exposed to a continuous barrage of news about layoffs, budget cuts, and the economic impacts of the pandemic. All that negativity can leave employees with feelings of impending doom - unsure about their jobs and their futures.

Negativity

The term *negativity bias* refers to our tendency to pay more attention to and fixate on the bad things in our life, which can further feed our insecurities. With negativity surrounding them, your remote employees may dwell on any negative feedback, negative comments, or something stupid they said in last week's meeting. Those insecurities and feelings of despair can result in depression and anxiety and negatively influence attitudes. They can also color interactions with coworkers and family.

A general sense of negativity is difficult to disguise and can unfortunately be spread throughout the organization—creating a culture of negativity. Emotional contagion is the phenomenon that individuals tend to express and feel emotions that mirror others around them. During the pandemic, your employees are surrounded by news about death, workforce reductions, business closings, and economic uncertainty. Those are bound to elicit negative feelings that can decrease motivation and job satisfaction and can easily be spread to others.

In a study (Grenny & Maxfield, 2017) of remote employees, they reported often feeling left out and even mistreated by their coworkers. They also indicated that they thought that other employees lobbied against them and talked about them behind their backs. Because they aren't in close proximity to other coworkers, it becomes easier for them to leave coworkers out of decisions. It also makes it more difficult to resolve those conflicts. Ongoing conflicts with coworkers can negatively influence morale and productivity.

Management Tips

While you are not going to be able to alleviate all employees' insecurities, there are things that can be done to avoid contributing to the problem. Be honest. Any employee, particularly those working remotely, will appreciate honesty and transparency—even when you have bad news. When employees don't get information about what is happening with the organization, they may concoct their own versions. With a general sense of doom or a negative attitude, those employee versions are likely to be worse than the reality.

- Work to avoid negativity and negative comments.
- Practice positivity.
- Encourage employees to seek out positive relationships with coworkers.
- Be honest and transparent.
- Work to create a shared purpose.
- Review and revise existing workflows for maximum transparency.

Remote management skills required: communication, connection.

REMOTE WORKFORCE MANAGEMENT SKILLS

The pandemic has, for many, necessitated a new way to work. Issues relating to remote work environment, isolation, insecurity, and work boundaries can combine to contribute to both mental and physical exhaustion for your remote employees. Consider that many workers lucky enough to still have jobs, have been required to work remotely for more than a year - far longer than they anticipated. Reflect on the issues that were discussed here and you can see how their motivation, dedication to the organization, and productivity might suffer.

In response to this new way of working, managers need a new way to manage. As mentioned throughout the chapter, there are things you can do to understand, motivate, and manage your remote workforce more effectively. Take the time to talk to your employees and work to really connect with them. Allow for some one-on-one time because they may be hesitant to share their struggles in front of coworkers. It may be the only way

Figure 13.2

Remote Workforce Management Skills

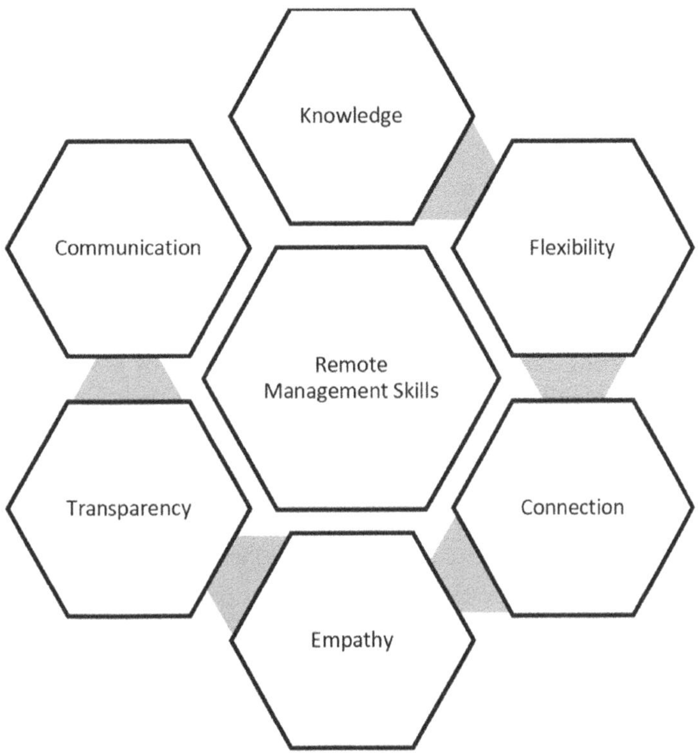

you will discover what specific issues they are dealing with. After all, you will struggle to help them, if you do not understand what they need.

For a good manager, these are not new skills, but they can be utilized in new ways to help address the unique needs and concerns of your employees who are working remotely. These skills center around six broad categories: knowledge; flexibility; connection; empathy; transparency; and communication (see Figure 13.2).

Knowledge

There are some new things you should know when managing employees who work off site. Remote employees, particularly those who are using their own computers or unsecured networks, present some new concerns surrounding information security. Familiarize yourself with the data access permissions your employees have and limit access to sensitive data, if possible. It is important for you to also be familiar with basic data security measures that are available, such as virtual private networks and videoconference settings that ensure privacy. Also, regardless of whether you have human resources professionals in your organization, you should be familiar with new employment and tax laws and how they apply to your organization.

Flexibility

Work to be as flexible as possible with work assignments, which will help employees who are struggling with balancing work with family responsibilities. While some managers may be reluctant to allow such autonomy, setting clear guidelines and expectations for performance can help. If possible, allow employees to complete work assignments when it is convenient for them, but be specific about the quantity of work and assignment deadlines. Be flexible when it comes to meetings too. Allow your employees to keep cameras off if it makes them more comfortable and specify which meetings are mandatory and which might be optional. Scheduling fewer meetings can help alleviate anxiety about the noise and condition of their work environments.

Connection

Connecting with your employees becomes very important when they are working remotely. They need to be informed and feel connected to perform at their best. Be strategic about how you communicate with them and make time for socialization and personal connections. However, remember that there's a delicate balance between too much and not enough. Make your connections count. Excessive or unnecessary virtual meetings result in a drain on your employees' time—time that they could use to be productive. Also, avoid texting or emailing employees outside of work hours, if possible and be specific about when employees should be available. Remote employees often struggle with the ability to disconnect from work. It does not help when they feel like they have to check for communication around the clock.

Empathy

In the present environment, your remote employees are likely to be struggling with any number of issues simultaneously. Empathy, understanding the feelings of others, is especially important during this time.

Developing and showing empathy toward all of your employees can help build camaraderie and a sense of team. Listen carefully to what they say and pay attention to their emotional state. Without empathy, your employees can feel unappreciated and even more disconnected from the organization. In addition, misunderstandings and conflicts are certain to escalate. Work to understand and offer support and encouragement to those who are struggling. It may you feel better too.

Transparency

As they struggle with insecurities, your remote workforce needs honesty and transparency from you. When working remotely and autonomously, information silos can occur, preventing employees from access to information they need to be productive. Consider evaluating existing workflows and make them more transparent. Also, especially while in the wake of the pandemic, you will undoubtedly be faced with making unpopular decisions, disseminating discouraging news, or even reducing the size of workforce. Your employees understand that. Being honest and transparent can help reduce gossip and spreading of misinformation among your employees. It can also help alleviate feelings of insecurity and disconnection.

Communication

When your employees work remotely, communication becomes the only way they remain connected to your organization. Keeping them informed is critical but avoid utilizing too many delivery modes. Your employees can get frustrated or miss important information if they're forced to search for it in more than one location. Avoid information overload by working to summarize information, if you can, rather than inundating your employees with emails every time you have a new thought or scheduling unnecessary videoconferences. Finally, try to limit communications to business hours, which can help remote employees maintain boundaries between work and home.

CONCLUSION

Working from home or other remote locations during the pandemic may have been a new way of doing things for many of us. Having a workforce dispersed geographically also presents a host of new struggles for them. In fact, for managers and employees alike, it is whole new ball game—one that is not likely to change soon. Now that many organizations have seen that it can be done effectively and often with a significant cost savings due to a reduced need for space and equipment, it's clear that remote work is here to stay. Consequently, learning to understand the unique struggles of remote employees will help you to motivate and manage them to perform their best. Incorporating the skills of knowledge, flexibility, connection, empathy, transparency, and communication into your management toolbox can only serve to benefit you, your workforce, and your organization. After all, regardless of how and where you believe you'll be working in the future, we never know what lies around the corner.

REFERENCES

Benson, J. A., McSorley, V. E., Hawkley, L. C., & Lauderdale, D. S. (2021). Associations of loneliness and social isolation with actigraphy and self-reported sleep quality in a national sample of older adults. *Sleep: Journal of Sleep and Sleep Disorders Research*, *44*(1), 1–9. https://doi.org/10.1093/sleep/zsaa140

Bucurean, M. (2020). The impact of working from home on productivity. A study on the pandemic period. *Annals of Faculty of Economics, 1*(12), 267–275.

Buffer. (2021). *State of remote work 2019*. https://buffer.com/state-of-remote-work-2019

Burroughs, A. (2020). Adapting to change: Recognize employees' needs as they adjust to remote work. *Smart Business Pittsburgh*, *27*(7), 10–10.

Centers for Disease Control and Prevention. (2020a, November 4). Loneliness and social isolation linked to serious health conditions. https://www.cdc.gov/aging/publications/features/ lonely-older-adults.html

Centers for Disease Control and Prevention. (2020b). Cited in Understanding the effects of social isolation on mental health. Tulane University, School of Public health and Tropical Medicine, December 8. https://publichealth.tulane.edu/blog/effects-of-social-isolation-on-mental-health/

Csercevits, J. (2021, April 21). Trade secret protection with a remote workforce: 7 practical considerations for employers. *JD Supra*. https://www.jdsupra.com/legalnews/trade-secret-protection-with-a-remote-7257867/

Chapman, B., Swainston, J., Grunfeld, E. A., & Derakshan, N. (2020). COVID-19 outbreak effects on job security and emotional functioning amongst women living with breast cancer. *Frontiers in Psychology*, *11*. https://doi.org/10.3389/fpsyg.2020.582014

Chekwa, C. (2018). Don't be left out—Fostering networking opportunities to reduce workplace isolation among ethnic employees in remote settings. *Journal of Competitiveness Studies*, *26*(3/4), 217–235.

Huang, Y., & Chang, C.-H. (Daisy). (2020). Supporting interdependent telework employees: A moderated-mediation model linking daily COVID-19 task setbacks to next-day work withdrawal. *Journal of Applied Psychology*, *105*(12), 1408–1422. https://doi.org/10.1037/apl0000843

Garrison, M. (2021). *Legal issues to consider when transitioning to a remote workforce*. Nolo.Com. https://www.nolo.com/legal-encyclopedia/legal-issues-to-consider-when-transitioning-to-a-remote-work- force.html

Gorlick, A. (2020, March 30). The productivity pitfalls of working from home in the age of COVID-19. *Stanford News*. https://news.stanford.edu/2020/03/30/productivity-pitfalls-working-home-age-covid-19/

Grenny, J., & Maxfield, D. (2017). A study of 1,100 employees found that remote workers feel shunned and left out. *Harvard Business Review Digital Articles*, 2–5.

Hickman, A. (2019, November 6). *How to manage the loneliness and isolation of remote workers*. Gallup. https://www.gallup.com/ workplace/268076/manage-loneliness-isolation-remote-workers.aspx

Hinds, P., & Elliott, P. H. (2021, February 9). *Viewpoint: Why remote work doesn't have to dilute your company's culture*. SHRM. https://www.shrm.org/resourcesand-tools/hr topics/technology/pages/ viewpoint-why-remote-work-doesnt-have-to-dilute-your-companys-culture.aspx

Johanson, M. (2021, February 22). *How your space shapes the way you view remote work*. https://www.bbc.com/worklife/article/20210218-how-your-space-shapes-the-way-you-view-remote-work

Jung, H. S., Jung, Y. S., & Yoon, H. H. (2021). COVID-19: The effects of job insecurity on the job engagement and turnover intent of deluxe hotel employees and the moderating role of generational characteristics. *International Journal of Hospitality Management*, *92*, 102703. https://doi.org/10.1016/j.ijhm.2020.102703

Koslowski, N., Linehan, C., & Tietze, S. (2019). When is a bed not a bed? Exploring the material and virtual in negotiating home-work boundaries. *Culture and Organization*, *25*(3), https://doi.org/10.1080/14759551.2017.1349128

Kurowska, A. (2020). Gendered effects of home-based work on parents' capability to balance work with non-work: Two countries with different models of division of labour compared. *Social Indicators Research*, *151*(2), 405–425. https://doi.org/10.1007/s11205-018-2034-9

Lando, P. (2020, December 2). *Practical guidance on protecting trade secrets while working remotely*. https://www.entrepreneur.com

Lobell, K. O., & Lobell, K. O. (2020, July 30). *Accommodating working parents during the COVID-19 Pandemic*. SHRM. https://www.shrm.org/resourcesandtools/hr-topics/employee-relations/pages/accommodating-working-parents-during-the-covid-19-pandemic.aspx

Lowy, J. (n.d.). Overcoming remote work challenges. *MIT Sloan Management Review*. https://sloanreview.mit.edu/article/overcoming-remote-work-challenges/

Lufkin, B. (n.d.). What happens when you work from bed for a year. https://www.bbc.com/worklife/article/20210217-is-it-bad-to-you-work-from-your-bed-for-a-year

McLay, L., Jamieson, H. A., France, K. G., & Schluter, P. J. (2021). Loneliness and social isolation is associated with sleep problems among older community dwelling women and men with complex needs. *Scientific Reports*, *11*(1), 1–10. https://doi.org/10.1038/s41598-021-83778-w

Mercado, D. (2020, September 23). Grappling with childcare while working from home? How employers plan to help. *CNBC*. https://www.cnbc.com/2020/09/23/dealing-with-childcare-while-working-at-home-how-employers-will-help.html

Modi, A. (n.d.). The untold side of remote working: Isolation and lack of career progression. *Forbes*. https://www.forbes.com/sites/ankurmodi/2019/12/26/the- untold-side-of-remote-working-isolation-and-lack-of-career-progression/

Moss, J., & Moss, J. (2020, April 25). Dealing with social isolation. *SHRM*. https://www.shrm.org/hr-today/news/all-things-work/pages/dealing-with-social-isola- tion-due-to-coronavirus.aspx

National Law Review. (2021, April 24). *Protecting trade secrets while employees work remotely*. https://www.natlawreview.com/article/tools-used-modern-business-such-videoconferencing-and-social-media-culture-create

Nedelcu, E. (2020). The perspective of young people on the effects of telework on the quality of life at work. *Romanian Review of Social Sciences, 19*.

Ozcelik, H., & Barsade, S. G. (2018). No employee an island: Workplace loneliness and job performance. *Academy of Management Journal, 61*(6), 2343–2366. https://doi.org/10.5465/amj.2015.1066

Parker, S. K., Knight, C., & Keller, A. (2020, July 30). Remote managers are having trust issues. *Harvard Business Review*. https://hbr.org/2020/07/remote-managers-are-having-trust-issues

Rocco, P. (2020). Let me go to the office! An investigation into the side effects of working from home on work-life balance. *International Journal of Public Sector Management, 33*. https://doi.org/10.1108/IJPSM-06-2020-0150

van der Lippe, T., & Lippényi, Z. (2020). Beyond formal access: Organizational context, working from home, and work–family conflict of men and women in European workplaces. *Social Indicators Research, 151*(2), 383–402.https://doi.org/10.1007/s11205-018-1993-1

Westfall, C. (n.d.). Statistics show remote workers are frustrated, many still unprepared for working from home. *Forbes*. https://www.forbes.com/sites/chriswestfall/2020/08/25/statistics-show-remote-workers-are-frustrated-many-still-unprepared-for-working-from-home/

CHAPTER 14

MEASURING SUCCESS DURING A PANDEMIC

Time Management, Mindfulness, and Staying Positive

Kimberly Castle

> "Once the storm is over, you won't remember how you made it through, how you managed to survive. You won't even be sure the storm is over. But one thing is certain. When you come out of the storm, you won't be the same person who walked in."
>
> —-Haruki Murakami

INTRODUCTION

On March 11, 2020, the World Health Organization declared the world to be in a health pandemic. The COVID-19 pandemic caused enormous disruption in businesses. It will take years to recover from this disruption, and it likely to lead to the permanent shut down of many businesses that have been unable to bear the unprecedented difficulties and financial losses caused by the pandemic (Guleria & Kaushik, 2020). At this writing,

Back to a New Normal: In Search of Stability in an Era of Pandemic Disruption—Insight From Practitioners and Academics, pp. 201–213

according to the Small Business Administration, we are in the midst of a pandemic, one year in, and the number of small businesses open is down 34% (2021). According to the Centers for Disease Control and Prevention (CDC), since COVID-19, anxiety and depression is up 41% in working adults (2021). If businesses survived, they found ways to work differently—with options of remote work or working in shifts so that social distancing remained possible. Many industries found themselves working from home for the first time ever. Whether one is going to work or working remotely, the COVID-19 pandemic has likely changed the way we work (Centers for Disease Control and Prevention, 2020). Emotional distress, logistical challenges and time management have all played a role in this new reality. Success will look different postpandemically.

Companies are trying to administratively run from a "work from home mode" caused by the rigid requirements announced by Federal and State governments during COVID-19. Prior to COVID-19, most of those jobs from our home offices were limited to information technology or customer service. Now, many sectors of business have adapted to remote work business practice. One study by Guleria and Kaushik (2020) focused on work-life balance during this crisis of social isolation and distancing. They found that many folks were experiencing anxiety and, to overcome these emotional concerns, it is helpful to deploy positivity and routine so that the delicate work-life balance can achieve some semblance of normalcy (2020).

Working from a home office during a pandemic or unexpected crisis presents unique challenges and conflicts. Some of the challenges center around time management because of the other duties that we are responsible for in our homes—things like laundry, cooking, pet care, or childcare. Other challenges center on deadlines and the expectations that other members of our work team have as we work remotely. Being mindful about scheduling, priorities, and others' distractions helps when communication is limited due to a remote work environment. We have come to appreciate how emotional distress may creep into our lives at such a time, intensified by possible isolation.

Ultimately, staying positive and focusing on the tasks at hand may help us as we build these remote skills into our daily plans. It is fair to say we have never had to work through a pandemic before, and dramatic change is almost always met with some conflict. By mindfully and strategically planning our workdays from home, we may achieve our goals and maintain our equilibrium.

Since remote work during a pandemic such as COVID-19 is happening on platforms where there is in turn an unusual level of uncertainty and confusion, work can be interrupted by distractions, the news media, politics, and other factors that strain our sensibilities. Managing our time effectively and being mindful of tasks and our emotional reactions can also help us achieve success in uncertain times. This chapter will focus on time management, mindfulness, and positivity as key factors that can aid us in times of crisis.

TIME MANAGEMENT

If the term, time management, is googled, it pops up with over 97,000 finds. Perhaps that is because we all want more time, time to get the job done well, time to live longer when we get news of an illness, time to spend with those we care about, time to make up when we made a mistake, time for that lost goal, etc. The importance of time is immeasurable. COVID-19 has caused many of us to evaluate our time differently. For example, being blessed with a job we love, may make us grateful for our work time; on the other hand, being cursed with a job we dislike, may cause us to look for a better job. When the order to stay home challenged an entire country to do just that, the uncertainty of it all caused great worry about time and money. Money and time are often linked in conversation and writings. Benjamin Franklin (1748) had a saying, "Time is money." That rings true today as we measure success by how much money we save, or how large our salaries may be, or how time spent on anything minor might be considered, time wasted. For practical purposes, working from home has caused us to reconsider how we spend and budget our time given our greater immersion in work.

From the time we are school-age, we are taught to tell and value time. We take timed tests, we follow schedules when we change class, and even lunchtimes and recesses are budgeted into the school day equation based upon a limited number of hours in a day. Unknowingly, we begin managing time from when we are quite young. It becomes even more important as we become working adults. Eventually, we mature and plan our own time. "Managing" our time takes on even greater meaning. Management implies control, maintaining order, and being effective. Thus, managing our time, suggests that, if we do not manage time, someone else might or we might fail. Both can be scary prospects. One certainty about our time during uncertain times is that time is a valued asset.

For many of us, a home workspace is an area or room repurposed to allow for some remote computer work, undisturbed by other activity in our homes. At an early point during this author's work, each adult son was on zoom school in adjoining rooms, and we could all hear one another. We therefore adjusted and accommodated by getting personal headphones and closing doors. We learned to adjust and compromise by communicating when each of us needed a quiet space. We had to suspend the family considerations and behave more like a work team in order to share workspace and work productively during these unprecedented times.

We spend an estimated 43% of our working day, whether on worksite or at home, doing things without thinking consciously about them, This means that we do many things as a result of our sub-conscious mind nudging our body to act along learned behaviors (Wood, 2020). Further, COVID-19 has affected everyone as the global pandemic triggered a surge of stress hormones for example, adrenalin and cortisol, which can cause dramatic behavior changes—in some, to lose weight, finish a degree, pay down debt, or improve sleep habits and relationships—in others, to gain weight, watch TV, create more debt, spend more online, stay up late and vent emotionally or pull away from others (Wood, 2020). James Clear (2018) says, "Time magnifies the margin between success and failure and will multiply whatever you feed it. Good habits make time your ally and bad habits make time your enemy." Time management matters.

Time management is one of the most common factors affecting productivity under normal circumstances, let alone more stressful times like during a pandemic. Negative side effects of remote work are that we may get disengaged from work associates or our supervisors, or our workday may get filled with interruptions such as a ringing doorbell, preparing meals, laundry, internet issues, et cetera. Since schools have largely not been in person, children are typically at home on their zoom schools, which may require supervision. Additionally, without that in-person connection with work, it may make us feel disconnected from the organization (Guleria & Kaushik, 2020). Due to that lack of connection, there is a heightened retention challenge for many organizations (2020). Under these circumstances, we may revert to being very focused or we may procrastinate more. Ground rules can help. While researching this chapter, the author encountered many partially conducted studies as this subject matter is fairly new. However, as an old school author, when examining time management, it helps to be reminded of some basic principles that are mostly applicable:

1. Create a workspace that is your own—whether a kitchen table, a spare bedroom, or a large closet. clear it and make it neat and tidy and equipped for work (*Forbes*, *Good Housekeeping*, CDC, etc., 2020). A neat and tidy workspace is more productive (2020).
2. Start the day early, as a normal workday, treating our home office professionally helps productivity (*Goldman*, 2021).

3. Take scheduled breaks. According to *MacArthur* (2020), clocking more hours is easy to do because working from home means work is always calling.
4. Get good at setting and managing boundaries. Remember, there is a work team and a home team when working from home and sharing living space with spouses, children, pets, or roommates. This means that discussions about work times must be met with an inclusive mind. Normally, we do not check with our children when attending a zoom meeting, but if they are on zoom that needs simultaneous supervision, stress or unexpected developments may occur (MacArthur, 2020). Everyone is in the same boat, so inform your workplace when a challenge arises and work as a team. This may seem like your time is not always your own. Setting boundaries does not mean we cannot be flexible, but it keeps our time respected. Golden (2021) also recommended setting limits on household noise and having ground rules for household members concerning expectations so that boundaries are respected.
5. Be your own empowered spokesperson. Keep in touch with coworkers and let them know what you are working on and your progress; in other words, toot your own horn! Since working from home does not foster communication and kinship with a company, a lack of psychological association with the company might be present. Assert yourself and this may help reduce low reliability or retention worries felt by employers (Golden, 2021). This may also ensure that your employer has direct accountability for your work so that there is less needless interaction about whether or not we are on task.

A study published by Rensselaer Polytechnic Institute (Gallagher, 2021) before the onset of Coronavirus indicates that those who work from home regularly while eligible to be considered for promotions are likely to suffer from overall lower pay increases than those given to on-premises employees. Some of the challenges that we are seeing now stem from employers that typically do not support a geographically dispersed workforce. Managers and supervisors may be ill-equipped to manage staff remotely. In general, management style and culture are deeply ingrained and tend to fit into either the McGregor Theory X or Theory Y model. "X" management believes that workers need to be closely watched to keep them on task, while "Y" management believes that if you hire the right people and give them the tools that they need, they will invariably do the right thing. The "Y" style conveys a culture of trust, and trust is the key ingredient for success in the current circumstances (Golden, 2021). Certainly, as employers and employees are both working remotely, measuring success, and accountability might need to be adjusted for more meaningful ways of looking at success. If we manage our time wisely as we work remotely in a time of crisis, both the employee and the employer can reap success! Even if we do our best, crisis may still cause high stress and lead to burnout. However, we can learn even from failure and move forward.

BURNOUT

Hines (2020) defines burnout as a state of emotional, mental, and often physical exhaustion brought on by prolonged or repeated stress. Further, the Hines states that it is often caused by problems at work, but it may also appear due to parenting, relationships, caretaking, or other stressful developments in our lives. Hines (2020) says that burnout refers specifically to phenomena in the workplace context and should not be applied to describe experiences in other areas of life (2019). Hines (2020) further claims that burnout leads to the following:

- feelings of energy depletion or exhaustion,
- increased disconnection from one's job, or feelings of negativism or cynicism related to one's job, and
- reduced professional efficacy.

Without effective time management, burnout is a possibility as challenges around the unknown may take a toll on us as we work from home. Self-care is sometimes thought to be selfish, but research shows it is necessary (Barth, 2019). Self–care encourages us to maintain a healthy relationship with ourselves so that we can transmit positive feelings to others. We cannot give to others what we do not have ourselves. Authors like Brene' Brown have cited massive amounts of research that support this critical idea. Specifically, she writes about vulnerability and the good that comes from it (2012). She further says that "during these trying times, families need a plan" and in an emergency, for instance we "all handle it differently" for example the coronavirus outbreak (2020). She further states, "I think collectively what I see is a growing weariness. I think we are tired—physically, emotionally, and spiritually exhausted" (Brown, 2012). Brown explained that we all have enough adrenaline to get through short-lived crises, but this pandemic is not short-lived (2020). Managing our expectations can help us overcome the burnout we may experience. Recognizing this possibility will also enable us to overcome burnout by helping us build self-care into our time management routines.

MINDFULNESS DURING A CRISIS

A technique used to prevent or manage burnout is mindfulness. The term, mindfulness is no longer just a buzzword in management science. Mindfulness began over 2,500 years ago as a part of Buddhism (Langer, 1989). Stay mindful of the things that lead to negativity and steer clear—when negative thoughts enter our minds, and be prepared to change course (Castle, 2020). Being mindful means that we take active steps to solve problems and we do not give in to the need to win or the need to control—we try to remain neutral, proactive, and thoughtful at every turn (Castle, 2020). By keeping our thoughts positive, we can focus on the task at hand and not the larger universe. The law of attraction teaches us that positive thinking breeds positivity and negative thoughts breed negativity.

The *Harvard Business Review* researched the effectiveness of mindfulness at work, and they found that mindfulness helps build resilience and decreases the effects of anxiety and stress. Further, it was discovered that mindfulness enhances our ability to perform under stress. Research has also shown that our brains are changed when we apply mindfulness towards better decision-making skills (Congleton et al., 2015). By simply taking two minutes for deep breathing and meditation, we can improve our ability to act calmly and cope with things that come into our workday path (2015). Empirical research suggests that mindfulness fosters greater insight and more "out of the box" innovative thinking (Birk, 2020).

Mindfulness helps us with creativity, our focus, and our interpersonal relationships (Birk, 2020). Techniques toward mindfulness include meditation. We are all guilty of occasionally working on autopilot and, when distractions occur, it can be hard to stay on task (2020). Mindfulness teaches us how to live in the here and now. When we meditate and take a scheduled break from our work and place our minds in a calm, relaxing place, we return to our work refreshed, according to research (2020). Being mindful is staying in the moment and remaining focused on the here and now. Mindfulness can be learned. There are mindful apps on our phones that we can download and use to learn these techniques. Common steps to take toward becoming mindful include being aware of your surroundings, breathing deeply, meditating, and practicing gratitude.

Mindfulness management helps with patience, communication, and relaxation especially before tense meetings or deadlines. Furthermore, mindfulness keeps us "in the moment" and less distracted. It is also a technique that leads to positivity.

POSITIVITY DURING TIMES OF CRISIS

A 2011 report published in *Applied Psychology: Health and Well-Being* (Deiner & Chan, 2011) examined the effects of well-being and how people sum up their own lives, and the report concluded that happiness could influence health. The report looked at subjective areas of well-being such as judgments on life satisfaction and other emotional reactions (Chopik et al., 2011). Further, when people feel a sad mood or a joyful emotion, it is due they believe to their lives going badly or well (Chopik et al., 2011). It sounds simple but those words mean different things to each of us based upon our lived experiences, conflicts, and values. Realizing that we all come from varying perspectives, the report offered some interesting theories such as:

1. Happy people take better care of themselves—it makes sense that when we are more happy than sad, we make positive choices.
2. Happy people choose healthy behaviors, like exercising, eating well, and getting good sleep—it makes sense to promote continued positive feelings.

Imagine that—we are happy if we are healthier, and the report shared that there is likely a link between psychological well-being, aging and health (MacMillan, 2021). Being happy does not ensure better health, but evidence suggests there is a strong connection. According to Harvard research (Kubzansky et al., 2019), the more optimistic people are, the longer they live. Further, pessimism is linked to poor health (2019). The same research also concluded that the optimist also reports less stress, and the self-proclaimed optimist had fewer cardiac health issues (2019). Studies also show that optimists have longer-lasting, deeper, and more supportive relationships, and they are better at solving problems with friends and loved ones too (Chopik, 2020).

So, how do we advance positivity? We feed it. There is an old saying that states, "That which controls our thoughts, controls us." In the cycle of conflict, our lived experiences control our feelings (Castle, 2020), so by applying that idea to the goal of happiness, managing our thoughts makes sense. Real-world optimism techniques might help us achieve a more positive outlook. Below are some suggestions on how to gain a positive attitude and perspective.

1. Play your favorite inspirational music; this offers us warmth and often reminds us of a hopeful or happy time.
2. As with mindfulness, practice gratitude; look at a negative event as a path to something better.

3. Schedule time to grieve or worry; try not to feel that way outside of the ten minutes allotted daily.
4. Visualize your positive role model; imagine matching that positivity.
5. Visualize the end goal; think of setbacks as growth opportunities.
6. Speak positively; giving voice to negativity negates our way to positivity.
7. Be kind; treat others as we wish to be treated.
8. Be organized; neatness helps us organize our thoughts.
9. SMILE; Smiles are contagious, and they have the power to transform our outlook (Goldman, 2021). Masks have made it more difficult to discern another's smile. However, smiles can also be inferred through our eye contact, voice tone, and body language.

Happiness has linkages to the wellness movement (Hanson, 2013). People pursue happiness through activities such as taking CBD or essential oils, burning incense, acupuncture, cell phone detachment, forsaking sugars, and a myriad of other methods. Dr. Hanson's research concluded that having more inner strengths is a large key to a happy, productive, and loving life (2013). For example, his research shows that the inner strength of positivity reduces reactivity and stress (p. 6). Furthermore, positivity encourages us to seek opportunity, heal emotional wounds, and improve resilience (2013). During uncertain pandemic times, an optimistic outlook enables us to push on and weather the storm, so to speak.

Resilience is a component that allows humans to go on, even in traumatic times. Pandemics and times of crisis are surely traumatic. Many employers and employees have given interviews and written about turning off the television, being more introspective, and finding the inner strength to remain grateful and positive, using survival tactics, and continuing the path toward a thriving state of being. Staying positive and connected to loved ones may be the key to attaining resilience (Zaman, 2021). Resilience is defined as the ability to bounce back from adversity and misfortune. Resilience is an essential tool for being an effective leader (Ledesma, 2014). The literature demonstrates that there is a direct relationship between stress and the ability to maintain resilience in the face of prolonged exposure to adversity (2014). Variables found to be helpful for resilience and positivity include positive self-esteem, hardiness, strong coping skills, inner direction, self-efficacy, optimism, strong social resources, adaptability, risk-taking, low fear of failure, determination, perseverance, and a high tolerance for uncertainty (2014).

Two types of happiness, according to Hanson (2014), are hedonic and eudaemonic. Both are positive but different. Hedonic is a type of happy feeling stemming from a good fitting pair of jeans, or the first sight of a pink tree blooming overnight in spring—something brief and smile enhancing. Eudaemonic is a type of happy feeling that comes when we spend hours cleaning up after a storm and see the finished product, or when we sit with a friend in the emergency room for hours to provide emotional support—not necessarily fun happy but rewarding happy.

Hanson's research teaches us that there is no one way for being happy, but the ability to find joy over repeated episodes of happiness can help us to achieve a positive mindset. On average, about one third of our strengths (talents, skills, and personality traits) are innate—we are born with them; the other two-thirds, are developed over time, and "we acquire them through life experiences and growth" (Hanson, 2014). By working to achieve a positive mindset, engaging mindfulness and applying some of the steps above, we can experience positivity in the process!

> It is not the strongest of species that survive, nor the most intelligent, but the ones most resilient and responsive to change. —Darwin

SUCCESS

While working from home, implementing the techniques described above, namely time management, mindfulness, and positivity, we improve our prospects for success when we ultimately come out on the other side of this pandemic. With the right mindset, we can survive and thrive personally and professionally. Recently, a concept was presented at a training that impacted this author. When we think of a navy SEAL, the word, heroic or brave probably comes to the top of one's mind. There are positive and uplifting thoughts when we view the group as a team of problem solvers. If we all thought that way, it might look something like this (Sinicki, 2019):

Think like a navy SEAL:

1. Build resilience and mental toughness.
2. When you fall, get up again.
3. Ask for help.
4. Look for the good.
5. Ask who is a shining light during difficult times? And hang out with them!

During times of crisis and pandemics, if we all followed the Navy SEAL's way of thinking, how could we fail?

CONCLUSION

This chapter has provided insight into time management, mindfulness, and the use of positivity to overcome the negative aspects of a crisis or pandemic. By utilizing the tools learned above, one's toolbox becomes full of material to draw from when working from home to ensure the best experience for both the employee and employer who is navigating a crisis. Trying to implement all of these things at once can seem daunting. One is therefore advised to incorporate just one or two suggestions into one's daily toolbox and, upon success, implement a couple more, and so on.

Success is defined as achieving a desired outcome by *Webster's Dictionary* (online). Success may be one of those words that means something different to each of us. Elon Musk recently stated to *INC. Magazine Online,* that "failing at something means doing something wrong, or not being good enough. While at times, that may be true, failure is also a part of the journey to success" (Satara, 2018). Do not be afraid to fail. Walt Disney endured many failures before he went on to create the happiest place on earth. His autobiography (Krasniewicz et al., 2010) says he was rejected by banks over 300 times before one helped him with his Micky Mouse concept. He suffered a nervous breakdown and bankruptcy prior to achieving his dreams. Disney, like Elon Musk, has exhibited tenacity and persistence. Press on toward success and it can be attained. Remember, COVID will end, but the habits of resilience will live on.

REFERENCES

Barth, F. D. (2019, May 13). Self-care is important: Why is it so hard to practice? *Psychology Today*. https://www.psychologytoday.com/us/blog/the-couch/201905/self-care-is-important-why-is-it-so-hard-practice

Birk, M. (2020, November 20) Make mindfulness a habit. *Harvard Business Review Online*. www.hbr.org/2020/11/make-mindfulness-a-habit

Brown, B. (2012). The power of vulnerability: Teachings on authenticity, connection, and courage. *University of Houston Journal,* 1–45.

Castle, K. (2020). Manage anger spectrum pitfalls to work in your favor. In L. Wilkin & T. Belak (Eds.), *From discord to harmony: Making your workplace hum* (pp. 141–150). Information Age.

Centers for Disease Control and Prevention. (2021). CDC.gov. Retrieved February 2021.

Chopik, W., Oh, J., Kim, E., Schwaba, T., & Smith, J. (2020). Changes in optimism and pessimism in response to life events: Evidence from three large studies. *Journal of Research and Personality, 88*, 1–14.

Clear, J. (2018). *Tiny changes, remarkable results: Atomic habits*. Good Reads.

Congleton, C., Holzel, B., & Lazar S. (2015, January 8). Mindfulness can literally change your brain. *Harvard Business Review*. www.hbr.org/01/mindfulness-can-literally-change- your-brain.

Deiner, E., & Chan, M. (2011). Happy people live longer: Subjective well-being contributes to health and longevity. *Applied Psychiatry: Health and Well-Being, 3,*1–43.

Gallagher, J. (2021). How can remote workers best manage work-home conflict? *Rennsselaer News*. Online.

Golden, T. D. (2021). Telework and the navigation of work-home boundaries. *Organizational Dynamics, 50*(1), 1-10. 100822. https://doi.org/10.1016/j.orgdyn.2020
.100822

Goldman, L. (2021). The science of smiling: The power of positivits—A simple outlook can change your life. *Real Simple Magazine Special Edition*, 86–91.

Guleria, N., & Kaushik, M. (2020). The impact of pandemic Covid-19 in workplace. *European Journal of Business and Management, 12*(15), 9–18.

Hanson, R. (2013). *Hardwiring happiness: The new brain science of contentment, calm, and confidence.* Harmony Books.

Hines, R. (2020, March 30). Tensions running high at home? Try Brene' Brown's 'family gap plan.' Today.com. https://www.cdc.gov/coronavirus/2019-ncov/community/mental-health-non-healthcare.html

Krasniewicz, L., & Blitz, M. (2010). *Walt Disney: A biography*. Greenwood Biographies.

Kubzansky, L. D., David S., Pantel, V., & Kawachi, I. (2001). Is the glass half empty or half full? A prospective study of optimism and coronary heart disease in the normative aging study. *Psychosomatic Medicine, 63*(6), 910–916. https://doi.org/10.1097/00006842-200111000-00009

Langer, E. (1989). *Mindfulness*. Da Capo Press.

Ledesma, J. (2014). Conceptual frameworks and research models on resilience in leadership. *SAGE.open, 4*(3), 1–8. https://doi.org/10.1177/2158244014545464

MacArthur, H. U. (2020, April 4). Effective time management while working remotely during the COVID-19 pandemic. *Forbes Magazine Online*. https://www.forbes.com/sites/vickyvalet/2020/03/12/working-from-home-during-the-coronavirus-pandemic-what-you-need-to-know/?sh=158f19e11421

MacMillan, A. (2021, February 8). Happiness (probably) makes us healthier: While it certainly can't hurt, there is conflicting research on the link between mental and physical well-being. *Time Magazine*, 86–87. https://www.who.int/news/item/burn-out-an-occupational-phenomenon-international-classification-of-diseases

Satara, A. (2018, April 30). In 2 sentences Elon Musk explains why the key to success is failure. *Inc.* https://www.inc.com/alyssa-satara/in-2-sentences-elon-musk-explains-why-key-to-success-is-failure.html

Sinicki, A. (2019, December 31). Mental toughness: Think like a navy seal/spartan warrior. *The bioneer: Action, performance, technology.* www.thebioneer.com/mental-toughness-navy-seal/

Wood, W. (2020). *The science of making positive changes that stick: Good habits, bad habits*. Good Reads.

Zaman, M. (2021, February). What really makes us happy? *Time Magazine*, 42–45.

PART III

REMOTE LEARNING CHALLENGES AND CONSIDERATIONS

CHAPTER 15

ASYNCHRONOUS AND SYNCHRONOUS ONLINE LEARNING DURING A PANDEMIC

Anthony A. Piña

Throughout the 21st century, distance learning—and online learning in particular—has been the most consistent growth area within U.S. higher education. This has continued to be true, even during recent years of overall enrollment declines (Allen et al., 2016). The National Center for Education Statistics (2021) reported that in the 2018–19 year, 79% of U.S. degree granting institutions offered either standalone online courses or fully online programs and 56% offered both. This was especially pronounced at public colleges and universities, where 97% of 2-year and 96% of 4-year institutions offered some form distance learning.

The benefits afforded by online/distance education, include "anytime, anywhere" access and flexibility for students whose employment, family, health and/or other circumstances make adherence to traditional academic schedules and locations difficult or not possible. Higher education institutions can also benefit from increased enrollments and by offering their programs to students outside their traditional service areas (Clinefelter & Aslanian, 2015). This had led to online/distance education

Back to a New Normal: In Search of Stability in an Era of Pandemic Disruption—Insight From Practitioners and Academics, pp. 217–228

becoming institutionalized within numerous colleges and universities and an essential component of their strategic planning (Piña, 2008). A survey of chief academic officers at 2,807 postsecondary institutions indicated that more than 70% consider online education to be critical to their institution's long-term strategy, compared to less than 50% in 2002 (Allen & Seaman, 2015). Prior to the COVID-19 pandemic, it was estimated that more than 1/3 of postsecondary students in the U.S. were enrolled in at least one online course (National Center for Education Statistics, 2019a, 2019b; Seaman et al., 2018).

ONLINE AS A CONTINGENCY FOR CAMPUS CLOSURES

In the aftermath of the devastation of Hurricane Katrina in 2005, more than 120 universities provided thousands of tuition-free online courses to the students of over 20 colleges and universities that were forced to shut down (Meyer & Wilson, 2011; Schroeder, 2020). In addition to the threat of natural disasters, epidemics and pandemics—including SARS, Ebola, Zika, avian flu and swine flu—have led many institutions to adopt contingency plans for instances where campuses must close (Indiana State University, n.d.; McLennan, 2005; Meyer & Wilson, 2011).

> Unlike many other disasters which have the potential for destroying or disrupting a large portion of the university's infrastructure, a pandemic's greatest impact will be on personnel and absenteeism leaving our facilities largely untouched. Disruptions that do occur will result from insufficient numbers of personnel available to provide expected services. (Indiana State University, n.d., p. 1)

HIGHER ED INSTITUTIONS NOT WELL PREPARED FOR A PANDEMIC

In their analysis of 50 flagship universities, Meyer and Wilson (2011) noted that none stated an explicit policy or plan for delivering online courses in case of an emergency, instead offering suggestions to faculty for different options that they could consider. They concluded that these institutions were not well prepared and stated—prophetically—"One can expect more stories … as online learning and related technologies come to the aid of higher education institutions hit by various disasters in the future. And there will be more disasters" (p. 7).

Despite Schroeder's (2020) observation that lessons from Hurricane Katrina could help colleges and universities navigate the difficulties of the worldwide COVID-19 pandemic, it became clear that numerous colleges and universities had not fully institutionalized online learning across all programs and disciplines. As Meyer and Wilson (2011) had predicted nearly a decade earlier, when higher education institutions were compelled to shut down campuses and move their courses to fully online delivery in March of 2020, many were ill prepared for the challenge, as faculty training in online teaching and course development had largely been optional, with many faculty having opted out of the training (Garrett et al., 2020; Hodges et al., 2020).

EMERGENCY REMOTE TEACHING

Garrett et al. (2020) estimated that fully half of faculty faced with converting their courses from on-campus to online in March of 2020 had never previously taught an online course. Many of these faculty immediately began using online technologies (both synchronous and asynchronous) with little or no experience or training in their use. Given that online and face-to-face course development and teaching requiring different skill sets, it is unsurprising that many students and faculty would find teaching and learning under these conditions to be less than desirable (Hodges et al. 2020; Newsome et al., 2021).

Scholars and practitioners of online learning and teaching have expressed concern that the "emergency remote teaching" experienced by faculty and students in response to the pandemic would be confused with legitimate well-designed and well-taught online courses (Garrett et al., 2020; Hodges et al., 2020). As Hodges and his associates stated,

> Online learning carries a stigma of being lower quality than face-to-face learning, despite research showing otherwise. These hurried moves online by so many institutions at once could seal the perception of online learning as a weak option, when in truth nobody making the transition to online teaching under these circumstances will truly be designing to take full advantage of the affordances and possibilities of the online format. (Hodges et al., 2020, p.1)

ONE UNIVERSITY'S RESPONSE

Sullivan University is a privately owned, regionally accredited and doctoral granting institution with is main campus in Louisville, Kentucky. Sullivan University was founded in 1962 as an institution to meet the educational needs of working professionals and nontraditional students. Sullivan University began offering online courses in 2000, primarily to provide educational continuity for military students who were deployed to different parts of the country and the world.

In 2008, the university began to strategically build up its capacity and infrastructure for online learning by hiring instructional designers, establishing minimum quality standards and templates for master online courses, and evolving the process for online course development. Over time, the role of faculty developing online courses shifted from "putting their courses online" to being subject matter experts, working in partnership with instructional designers to create master online courses that could be taught by multiple instructors. By freeing faculty of the burden of having to do the configuration of assignments, discussion boards, tests, grade books, formatting, content chunking and accessibility, course development time was reduced.

The shift in course development culture and emphasis on instructional design and standards-based course creation and evaluation, included having most new courses and programs being developed first online, then adapted to face-to-face and hybrid modalities (Piña & Moran, 2018). The result was that, by 2020, the majority of the university's courses and degrees were available fully online. The increased demand for online course sections meant that most of the faculty had received training and had gained experience teaching online courses.

In March 2020, when COVID-19 pandemic restrictions were enacted by the state, Sullivan University was entering its final exam week of the winter 2020 quarter (the university is on a four-quarter, rather than a two-semester annual calendar). Faculty who had been teaching on-campus courses, quickly shifted their final exams, papers, et cetera, to the university's Blackboard learning management system. University leadership then had 2 weeks to plan for the spring 2020 quarter.

Because the university had invested in a team of six experienced instructional designers and two instructional technologists, more than 100 course sections, not previously taught online, were quickly developed by the instructional design team, with grade books and assignments ready for student submissions and faculty training support was provided by the instructional technologists. The majority of the courses for the spring 2020 quarter were already available as fully online masters, with course content that could be taught "as is" or customized to instructor needs.

While nearly all courses were able to be taught completely online or via synchronous web conferencing, there were a limited number of courses that required student use of specialized equipment in laboratory or clinical in-person sessions. It was determined that these courses would have online didactic content for the first several weeks, with the lab/clinical on-campus sessions at the end of the quarter in classrooms with masks, social distancing, and staggered meeting times with no more than 10 occupants in a classroom or lab.

The provost asked all faculty—including those teaching sections that were already slated to be online—to utilize the university's synchronous web conferencing platform to hold weekly virtual office hours and to provide live virtual instructional sessions, recording the sessions for students who were unable to attend the live session. Faculty received training in the use of Collaborate web conferencing platform and in Panopto for recording and editing asynchronous video announcements and instruction. A website for faculty development and resources was established to house printed job aids and short tutorial videos on Blackboard Learning Management System, Collaborate and Panopto.

At the end of the spring 2020 quarter (March–June 2020), the students completed their course and instructor evaluations. The composite scores indicated an overall high level of student satisfaction and were nearly identical to those of the (pre-COVID) winter quarter. Students commented that the increased use of video and synchronous sessions by their instructors made a positive difference to their educational experience, despite the challenges of the pandemic. The high student satisfaction scores continued during the summer 2020 (June–September), fall 2020 (September–December) and winter 2021 (January–March) quarters. Thanks to a dozen years of planning and building an infrastructure for online learning, strong leadership and extra efforts by the faculty and instructional design team, Sullivan University was able to continue instruction uninterrupted throughout the pandemic crisis.

LESSON LEARNED FROM PAST CRISES

Ray Schroeder (2020) provided one of the earliest articles intended to provide guidance to institutions affected by COVID-19. He outlined strategies that institutions could use as a result of lessons learned during Hurricane Katrina:

1. Create the delivery framework:
    - Have a central communication site (campus webpage) for students, staff and faculty.
    - Create a course shell in the learning management system for every class offered on campus.
    - Populate those classes with rosters when the decision to move forward is made.

- Move syllabi, discussion board, faculty announcements, and other "basics" online as soon as possible.

2. Triage priorities and ledgering:
    - Identify first courses to be served (e.g., largest enrollment classes; senior seminars and capstone classes).
    - Establish a clear hierarchy for triage.
    - Create an action priority spreadsheet and ledger of who is doing what, where they are in the process, and when each task is estimated to be complete.
    - Keep the team in constant contact—this will require multiple paths of communication for concurrent messaging and keeping records of communication. Technologies can include Slack, Microsoft Teams, Zoom, email, text messaging, et cetera.
3. Staffing and support:
    - Supplement instructional design staff with select faculty members who are online champions and mentors.
    - Consider 12-hour shifts and consider scheduling conference call meetings with faculty between 6 A.M. and midnight.
4. Cooperate, collaborate, communicate:
    - Do not let perfection become the enemy of good.
    - Instructors must decide what can reasonably done to advance learning to achieve the established learning outcomes for each class (e.g., reordering or organizing materials in a different way to accommodate the unexpected closure of campus).
    - Contact faculty and experts at other locations to share resources and virtual guest lectures.

ASYNCHRONOUS ONLINE INSTRUCTOR ENGAGEMENT

One of the most widely cited and recognized theories in online/distance education is transactional distance, which states that in an online course, there is not just a physical distance between students and their instructor, but also a psychological distance (Moore & Kearsley, 2012). There are "transactions" that instructors can do to increase instructor presence in the course and decrease the psychological distance (Lowenthal & Dunlap, 2014). In their study of how best to evaluate faculty teaching asynchronous online courses, Piña and Bohn (2016) identified seven indicators of engaged online instructors:

1. Posting a brief biography to allow students to get to know the instructor better. While text-based announcements are still dominant, faculty are increasingly taking advantage of introductory videos that bring students into their office, homes or hobbies. This "humanizes" the instructor and can lessen transactional distance (Lowenthal et al., 2020).
2. Posting course announcements at least weekly. Gaudet (2016) suggested that instructors can use course announcements to maximize their presence by allowing themselves to be creative and personal—while still being professional—by using anecdotes and personal observations. Announcements also provide opportunities to highlight upcoming activities, assignments, student contributions and current events relevant to that week's/lesson's topics.
3. Logging into and monitoring the online course on a daily basis. This allows instructors to monitor student progress, check for student questions and messages, and to quickly identify technical issues with the course. It is also a tangible indicator of instructor presence.
4. Piña and Bohn (2016) found that responding to student inquiries was considered to be the most important indicator of online instructor quality and engagement (tied with instructor feedback below). Having an instructor respond within 1 day of the inquiry was deemed to be most desirable, with 2 days being acceptable.
5. Providing helpful feedback to student assignments. This was also seen as a critical indicator of quality and engagement. Feedback is most helpful when it is timely and includes constructive guidance and explicit expectations (Getzlaf et al., 2009). Kelly (2014) recommended that instructors start with a positive message and employ rubrics to help students focus their work. Instructors should also take advantage of annotation tools within the learning management system and consider using audio and/or video feedback, which has been found to increase instructor presence and the quantity of feedback provided to students (Olesova & Borup, 2016).
6. Moderating and participating in discussion boards. Many instructors mistakenly believe that online discussion boards are to be used exclusively for student-to-student interaction. Instructors' active participation in online class discussions are a powerful indicator of instructor presence and provides the instructor with opportunities to respond to students individually and collectively and to engage in teachable moments. Instructors can moderate discussions through the use of "leading" questions (Piña et al., 2015).

7. Grading assignments in a timely manner. Grading and feedback tend to be the most time-consuming tasks for the online instructor; however, students often require the feedback from prior assignments to allow them to properly improve and prepare for future assignments. The University of Wisconsin-Stout (n.d.) provides several tips for managing online grading, including keeping comments and commonly used feedback from previous courses and adapting them to new students; using rubrics to make grading easier and to clarify expectations for the student; establishing peer feedback activities; scheduling self-graded or shorter assignments after a long, complex assignment, to allow time and energy for grading the longer assignments properly. Instructors should schedule grading during times of day where they tend to be tired or fatigued.

SYNCHRONOUS ONLINE INSTRUCTOR ENGAGEMENT

The response to the COVID-19 pandemic included an unprecedented increase in the use of synchronous desktop videoconferencing (also known as web conferencing). Daily meeting participants of Zoom—the most widely used platform—grew a staggering thirtyfold, from 10 million users to 300 million, between December 2019 and April 2020 (Kalmykov, 2020). Other major platforms, such as Microsoft Teams, WebEx, Go-To-Meeting, Google Meet and Blackboard Collaborate also saw huge increases. Many faculty members, intimidated by the time, effort and expertise required to design and develop fully online courses, opted to hold their class sessions via videoconference and ramp up their use of virtual office hours. Videoconference became a primary component of the "nontraditional instruction" used by K–12 schools during the pandemic.

The College of Literature, Science, and the Arts at University of Michigan (2020), provided a number of guidelines for instructors to engage in while delivering synchronous online instruction:

1. Prerecord lectures, demonstrations, and presentations. Instructors can best utilize their live synchronous videoconference time for activities that require students' active participation, such as question-and-answer sessions, one-on-one feedback, small group discussions, or collaborative work. Lectures, demonstrations and presentations can be watched by students prior to the synchronous session.
2. Create a detailed agenda and share it with students. An agenda helps to keep instructors and students on task, reduces wasted or irrelevant time, and helps to assure that all intended topics are addressed.

3. Make transitions explicit. In the absence of physical transitions of moving into groups or coming back together, instructors can provide transitional pauses between different learning activities or discussion topics. This allows students to a few moments to process the previous activity or task and prepare for the next one.
4. Just as with on-campus, classes, synchronous instructional sessions should include *taking regular breaks* (e.g., 5 minutes for every 30 minutes of instruction) to provide students with the opportunity to get up, stretch, or use the restroom. Breaks will help reduce students' cognitive load and fatigue and increase endurance.
5. Provide active learning opportunities. In addition to instruct-to-student interaction, synchronous class sessions should times where students engage in peer-to-peer interaction. These activities may include peer-taught class segments, minicase studies, simulations, role plays, weekly collaborative journal entries, small group discussions in breakout rooms, or paired analysis of a lab or demonstration video. Active learning will not only help to maintain student interest but will also foster a community of learning.
6. Be more flexible on attendance requirements. If students have connectivity issues or other circumstances that cause them to miss a synchronous session, plan for a research assignment or another alternative to the live assignment. Sessions can also be recorded, with assignments based on either attending or viewing the recorded sessions.

RESOURCES FOR ASYNCHRONOUS AND SYNCHRONOUS ONLINE TEACHING

Soon after the COVID-19 pandemic began affecting schools, colleges and universities around the world, The Association for Educational Communications & Technology, the leading international professional association for instructional design and educational technology, asked its members to provide resources that it could share freely with educators. The result is a 20-page document, with links to more than 70 different asynchronous and synchronous teaching resources organized under the topics listed next. The document can be accessed at: https://www.aect.org/docs/HigherEd_Resources_Commentaries.pdf.

1. Communicating with Students:
    - Communication tools
    - Providing feedback and feedback tools

- Strategies and best practices for communicating with students

2. Delivering Content Online:
   - Digital tools for delivering online content
   - Digital platforms for delivering online courses
   - Guidance and resources for teaching online
   - Examples of online courses
   - Resources and support during the COVID-19 crisis
3. Ensuring Accessibility:
   - Introduction to online accessibility
   - Comprehensive online accessibility resources
   - Disability inclusion
4. Meaningful Discussions:
   - Strategies for facilitating meaningful discussions—Getting started
   - Strategies for facilitating meaningful discussions—Learning more
   - Digital tools for discussion
5. Online Tests and Assessments:
   - Strategies for online assessment
   - Open book exams
   - Digital tools for assessment

CONCLUSION

As with natural disasters and health crises in the past, advances in technology have been utilized to mitigate some of their negative effects. In the case of the COVID-19 pandemic, many colleges and universities that had previously rejected online learning found that asynchronous and synchronous online learning was key to institutional survival. It remains to be seen if higher education will take the lessons from Katrina and COVID-19 and better prepare itself for the next hurricane, tornado, earthquake, or pandemic.

REFERENCES

Allen, I. E., & Seaman, J. (2015). *Grade level: Tracking online education in the United States*. Babson Survey Research Group and Quahog Research Group.

Allen, I. E., Seaman, J., Poulin, R., & Straut, T. T. (2016). *Online report card: Tracking online education in the United States*. Babson Survey Research Group and Quahog Research Group.

Clinefelter, D. L., & Aslanian, C. B. (2015). *Online college students 2015: Comprehensive data on demands and preferences*. The Learning House and Wiley.

Garrett, R., Legon, R., Fredericksen, E. E., & Simunich, B. (2020). *CHLOE 5: The pivot to remote teaching in spring 2020 and its impact, the changing landscape of online education, 2020*. Quality Matters. https://qualitymatters.org/qa-resources/resource-center/articles-resources/CHLOE-project

Gaudet, M. (2016). *Using course announcements to maximize instructor presence*. University of New England. https://online.une.edu/blog/using-course-announcements-maximize-instructor-presence

Getzlaf, B., Perry, B., Toffner, G., Lamarche, K., & Edwards, M. (2009). Effective instructor feedback: Perceptions of online graduate students. *Journal of Educators Online, 6*(2).

Hodges, C. B., Moore, S., Lockee, B. B., Trust, T., & Bond, M. A. (2020, March 27). The difference between emergency remote teaching and online learning. *EDUCAUSE Review*. https://er.educause.edu/articles/2020/3/the-difference-between-emergency-remote-teaching-and-online-learning

Indiana State University (n.d.). *Indiana State University pandemic operations plan*. https://www2.indstate.edu/pubsafety/docs/Final%20Pandemic%20Plan.pdf

Kalmykov, M. (2020). *Web conferencing boom: COVID-19's effect on the video call market*. https://medium.com/swlh/web-conferencing-boom-covid-19s-effect-on-the-video-call-market-153adc2f9d1

Lowenthal, P. R., & Dunlap, J. C. (2014). Problems measuring social presence in a community of inquiry. *E-Learning and Digital Media, 11*(1), 20–31.

Lowenthal, P. R., Borup, J., West, R. E., & Archambault, L. (2020). Thinking beyond Zoom: Using asynchronous video to maintain connection and engagement during the COVID-19 pandemic. *Journal of Technology and Teacher Education, 28*(2), 1–9.

McLennan, K. L. (2006). Selected distance education disaster planning lessons learned from Hurricane Katrina. *Online Journal of Distance Learning Administration* 9(4). https://www.westga.edu/~distance/ojdla/winter94/mclennan94.pdf

Meyer, K. A., & Wilson J. L. (2011). The role of online learning in the emergency plans of flagship institutions. *Online Journal of Distance Learning Administration 14*(1).

National Center for Education Statistics. (2019a). *Fast facts: How many students take distance learning courses at the postsecondary level?* U.S. Department of Education. https://nces.ed.gov/fastfacts/display.asp?id=80

National Center for Education Statistics. (2019b). *Trend generator*. U.S. Department of Education. https://nces.ed.gov/ipeds/TrendGenerator/app/trend-table/2/42

National Center for Education Statistics (2021). *Distance education in college: What do we know from IPEDS?* U.S. Department of Education. https://nces.ed.gov/blogs/nces/post/distance-education-in-college-what-do-we-know-from-ipeds

Newsome, M. L., Piña, A. A., & Mollazehi, M. (2021). *One year on: A national study of undergraduates' satisfaction with forced online learning in Qatar*. Manuscript submitted for publication.

Olesova, L., & Borup, J. (2016). Using audio and video feedback to increase instructor presence in asynchronous online courses. In S. D'Agustino (Ed.), *Creating teacher immediacy in online learning environments* (pp. 235–251). IGI Global.

Piña, A. A. (2008). Factors influencing the institutionalization of distance learning in higher education. *Quarterly Review of Distance Education 9*(4), 427–438.

Piña, A. A. & Bohn, L. (2016). Assessing online faculty. In A. A. Piña & J. B. Huett (Eds.), *Beyond the online course: Leadership perspectives on e-learning* (pp. 317-330). Information Age.

Piña, A. A., Merrifield, H., & Curry, J. (2015, November). *Strategies for improving the quality of online discussions* [Paper presentation]. Kentucky Convergence Conference, Bowling Green, KY.

Piña, A. A., & Moran, K. A. (2018, October). *Changing course development culture to improve learning for all* [Paper presentation]. Association for Educational Communications and Technology, Kansas City, MO.

Schroeder, R. (2020, March 11). What Katrina taught us about online delivery. *Insider Higher Ed.* https://www.insidehighered.com/digital-learning/blogs/online-trending-now/what-katrina-taught-us-about-online-delivery

Seaman, J. E., Allen, I. E., & Seaman, J. (2018). *Grade increase: Tracking distance education in the United States*. Babson Survey Research Group. https://onlinelearningsurvey.com/reports/gradeincrease.pdf

University of Michigan. (2020). *Best practices for synchronous remote learning*. https://lsa.umich.edu/technology-services/news-events/all-news/teaching-tip-of-the-week/best-practices-for-synchronous-remote-learning.html

University of Wisconsin-Stout. (n.d.). *Time management strategies for online instructors.* https://www2.uwstout.edu/content/profdev/rubrics/time_management.html

CHAPTER 16

THE MECHANICS OF REMOTE WORKING AND REMOTE LEARNING

A Logistics Perspective

Tom Javarinis

Since the first case of SARS-CoV-2 (also known as COVID-19 or coronavirus) was discovered on January 20, 2020,[1] life as we knew it turned upside down. Seemingly overnight, schools closed and went online, workplaces went remote, nonessential businesses were shuttered, and statewide lockdowns were imposed. People were—and are—fearful of the novel coronavirus that has currently taken the lives of over 500,000 Americans[2] and has caused the United States to enter into an economic recession. The impact of COVID-19 has been felt across all sectors, but it especially has been felt in academia. In Michigan, Governor Gretchen Whitmer suspended all in-person K–12 instruction for the rest of the 2019–2020 school year[3] and universities quickly followed suit, moving all instruction online. As of the writing of this chapter, 97% of Michigan K–12 schools met the criteria to open schools for in-person instruction.[4]

Like its K–12 counterpart, universities and colleges have also been affected by COVID-19. Many higher learning institutions also closed their

Back to a New Normal: In Search of Stability in an Era of Pandemic Disruption—Insight From Practitioners and Academics, pp. 229–239

doors to in-person instruction in 2020. Sullivan University delayed the start of their spring semester to April 6 and only allowed students in classrooms to complete final exams or turn in final projects.[5] Currently, Sullivan University has moved to online only instruction with some in-person allowed for nursing clinicals.

The decision to move from in-person instruction to online instruction has not only sparked a fierce national debate for K–12 schools but for higher education as well. With how quickly schools shuttered, many schools—including universities and colleges—struggled to cobble together an online platform to teach students. Some universities with robust online presences, including Sullivan University, seamlessly moved to online only instruction.[6] In both situations, educators rose to the challenge and developed clever and innovative ways to teach and inspire their students.

COVID-19's societal disruption continues to be felt in higher education 1 year after the first case of COVID-19 was discovered in the United States. While universities and colleges have opened their doors again, a majority of classes still remain online. As a 15-year educator, I have the unique position of not only having my feet in both the in-person learning and online learning worlds, but I also completed my PhD online as well. Throughout this year, I have encountered difficult challenges, developed new strategies, and learned valuable lessons while navigating working from home during a pandemic. My hope is that these strategies, lessons, and tips can not only help future educators successfully work and teach during perilous times but help students learn during perilous times.

REMOTE WORKING IN PERILOUS TIMES

I first started teaching in 2006 at Davenport University. In those days, teaching was mostly done in-person and very little instruction was done online. I did not move to online instruction until the 2009–2010 school year. When I made the switch to online instruction, I found online teaching to be much more difficult than in-person learning. It was very impersonal as you could not upload videos or audio. It was strictly a learning management system. In 2009, Zoom had not been created and not many people had webcams for face-to-face interaction. To be frank, I did not care for online instruction as I liked being able to see my students and see, through their body language and facial expressions if they were able to understand my instruction. Online instruction did not allow me that opportunity and I had to rely on my students to reach out to me to let me know if they were struggling with the course material.

As much as I did not initially like online instruction, I knew it would be the way of the future. Even in 2009, schools were starting to make the push to online instruction as it was a way for the school to allow students from near and far to attend that school and learn and it allowed the school to hire instructors from different regions from the country and these instructors did not need to leave the comfort of their homes. Even though I lived in Michigan, I was able to teach at a number of schools outside of my home state thanks to online instruction. A lot of universities—including Sullivan University—started to prioritize online instruction and learning. By the time, the 2019–2020 school year started, Sullivan University's courses were about 90% online and 10% in-person. Online instruction was here to stay and revolutionized higher education.

For the next 10 years, I spent a majority of my academic career not only teaching online but also designing and developing courses at Sullivan University. Prior to the pandemic, my course load was 85% online instruction. Due to my extensive experience in online instruction and remote work, I have discovered there are at least five principles to make the move to remote work successful:

KEEP YOUR WORK LIFE AND HOME LIFE SEPARATE

This tip may seem obvious, but I cannot stress the importance of keeping your home life separate from your work environment. In pre-COVID-19 times, employees could keep the line between their "work life" and "home life" separate and defined. Employees could clock out and be able to leave their office space and go home, divorcing themselves from their workday and enjoy the sanctity of their home environment. However, with a majority of employees working from home, that once defined line has now become blurred and work life now bleeds over into the home life. So how can one separate their work life from their home life? I have found that there are three ways to keep the line defined:

I have discovered that it is important to keep set work hours. As an online instructor, my students hail from not only the United States but from other countries as well. In order to accommodate as many student's time zones as possible, I have set specific work hours. Monday through Friday I start work at 10:00 A.M. and finish between 6 P.M. and 7 P.M., depending on the amount of work that needs to be completed. I also take an hour lunch and take two 20-minute breaks. Students are free to contact me anytime between my working hours. Due to COVID-19, I have extended my work hours to Saturday between the hours of 9 A.M. to 12 P.M. in order to better accommodate students who may not have an opportunity to reach out during the week. Although I am online during this set time during the weekend, I have found that an average of 1–3 students reach out during my Saturday hours so it is unlikely that I will keep my Saturday working hours outside of the pandemic. However, even though I have Saturday office hours, I make sure I only keep to the 3-hour window and log off afterwards.

It is also important to set clear boundaries while working from home. Establish clear expectations with your family and your students or employees. My family understands that Monday through Friday from 10 A.M. to 6 or 7 P.M. is work time and I am not to be disturbed unless it is an emergency or it's time for lunch or a break. My students know what my office hours are (typically, my office hours are my work hours) as I make sure that they're posted in Blackboard and in the announcements. It is imperative that you remain firm about your boundaries. If you are able to (or if your company provides it), use a separate laptop for work. My employer, Sullivan University, provides their faculty with work laptops and I make sure to use that work laptop exclusively for teaching. If your company provides a work cell phone, use that work phone exclusively for work only and do not use it after your work hours. If your company does not provide a work phone, find another way to delineate work and personal calls and emails. I use my personal phone for personal and work communications. In order to separate the two, I use a different ringtone for work emails, and I do not read emails from that ringtone after my work hours are over. These methods help to create a sense of separation between my personal life and my professional life.

The final tip that I have found helps separate my work life from home life is to literally separate the two. Turning a room into an office helps reintroduce the physical distinction between work and home. While it may seem convenient to work in the living room where you spend time with your family, you are inadvertently blurring the line between work and home. Once you have worked in the living room long enough, your oasis of peace and relaxation is now associated with stress and anxiety. It is important to separate the two as your environment shapes your state of mind. When you were in school, where would be the best place to study? The library. Why? Usually, we associate the library with studying and learning so when we enter the library, our state of mind is geared toward studying. That same logic should also apply to a home office. A space should be created so our mind can associate this area with productivity and efficiency. As I have been remote working for over a decade, I have been able to create an office in my basement. Once my work hours are over, I leave the office and do not return until my next workday. This ensures I keep the rest of my house stress free from work and also enables my brain to associate my basement office with work. I also recognize that not everyone has the space for a completely separate office. In that case, it's still important to create a separate space for work. Separate an area of your home and use that exclusively for work. Using different décor there or physically separating the space by using furniture helps your brain associate that specific area with work. If multiple people are working at home or remote schooling, using noise-canceling headphones also helps to minimize distractions and keep your brain associated with work.

ESTABLISH A ROUTINE

Working from home requires establishing a routine and sticking to it. This tip may again seem obvious, but its importance cannot be emphasized enough. While it may initially be thrilling to work from home, once the initial excitement wears off it can be intimidating to create and maintain your own work routine. In order to maximize my productivity and to get in the mental zone for work, I have found that it is important to try and ease into the day, such as you would if you were going into the office. I have also found that in order to get into a positive headspace, I do not check any work emails and I try to not consume any media first thing in the morning. A 2017 study found that 46% of Americans check their phones before they even get out of bed,[7] either checking emails, scrolling social media, or reading articles. With how devastating the pandemic has been, I find it necessary for my mental health to not read any news articles first thing in the morning.

While it may be tempting to roll out of bed and start work, I have found the best solution is to try and mimic a routine that is similar to if I was actually going into work. Set an alarm clock, shower, eat breakfast, and get dressed. While you do not have to wear your work attire, you need to treat the day like any other day at the office and you certainly cannot wear pajamas to the office! It's important for your brain to associate your workspace with work and your brain will only do so once you have established a routine.

Once you've established a morning routine, establishing a to-do list during work hours is also important. As stated above, my work hours during the workweek are 10 A.M. to 6/7 P.M. Monday through Friday and 3 hours on Saturday (but the weekend hours are only due to COVID-19). At the beginning of the work week, I write up a to-do list and try to stick to that list as much as possible. While the list is not set in stone (if something pops up, I will adjust my to-do list accordingly) I try to stick to the list as closely as possible. For example: on Mondays and Tuesdays, I spend the majority of my day grading student papers and responses to Blackboard discussion questions. Wednesdays are slow days because the weekly discussion question is posted on Blackboard and my students are busy reviewing the question and crafting their responses. Thursdays and Fridays are for responding to student posts and asking follow up questions to help facilitate the academic discussion.

Establishing and keeping a routine for your work from home space helps to ensure that you maintain productiveness and efficiency during work hours. It is so easy for you to become your own worst enemy while working from home but establishing a routine that is as similar as possible to an in-office routine will help keep you efficient and productive during work hours.

CREATE A SENSE OF COMMUNITY

To those who have not worked from home before, remote work seemed to be a dream perk. Who would not want to work in their pajamas and be able to avoid the morning and afternoon commute? However, a recent study has found that the remote work dream has become a nightmare to many employees, with an astonishing 60% of those surveyed stating they do not like working from home.[8] Since the start of the pandemic, employee mental health has also taken a nose dive too, with 28% of surveyed employees reporting positive mental health.[9] It is not difficult to theorize why mental health decreased in the last year and it is important to acknowledge that people may be facing pressures at home, including caring for their children while schools are shut, worrying about employment, the health of their family and friends, and dealing with isolation and insecurity.

The isolation and insecurity has been one of the toughest parts of the lockdown for many people. While I have worked from home for many years, I still found the isolation to be very difficult. Instead of engaging with my colleagues and students face to face, I now have to see them through a screen.

Not engaging with my colleagues and students face to face has been one of the toughest challenges of this pandemic and I cannot imagine how tough it has been on my students. One of the strategies I have implemented is to be as accessible as possible to my students. I reach out to students weekly, inquire about their wellbeing, and try to engage in a conversation with them. If my students have questions, I try to respond to their questions as quickly as possible. I try to do as many Zoom meetings as possible so students can actually see me. I have also found that my students respond positively to motivational quotes posted in weekly announcements and in Blackboard discussion posts. Based on that positivity, I have rethought the way I grade my student's assignments. I now try to provide more in-depth positive feedback while at the same time addressing their weaknesses so my students can see that there is a light at the end of the tunnel.

I have also realized that empathy is an important concept in this pandemic as well, as it provides an essential tool in inclusiveness and creating a sense of community. With restrictions that require people to be as distanced as possible, I have found it to be important to create a sense of community among my students so they know they have someone in their corner who they can go to if life gets too hard. I post a weekly Blackboard discussion board where students can discuss nonacademic matters. This is where my students can vent about issues in their lives, express their fears, or talk about their challenges. Not only does this provide some emotional relief but it also provides a necessary dialogue where the instructor and the student can mentor each other. These are unprecedented times, and it is my job to help navigate my students through these murky waters with confidence.

COMMUNICATION AND TECHNOLOGY ARE KEY

COVID-19 decimated our normal channels of communication. Conversations that used to take place in person are now done through technology. Instead of being able to witness verbal and nonverbal cues, we now have to guess if the tone of an email is positive or negative. Instead of getting an answer to a question immediately by popping into an office, we now have to wait until a colleague reads the message. While communication was important prior to COVID-19, it is even more important now and it is easier than ever to communicate due to technological advances.

Communication is one of the most basic ways to be successful at remote working. I would even argue that it Is one of the essential building blocks of efficient remote working. For industries that rely mostly on face-to-face interaction, the move to socially distanced communication can be difficult and onerous. However, there are a few tips I have learned to help make communication more effective during remote work.

Check in Often. While email may be the first thought for communicating, it's actually one of the many tools we now have in our toolbox to communicate more efficiently. Consider using video conferencing platforms instead like Zoom, Google Meet, or Skype. Having meetings via video conferencing can also stave off loneliness and isolation. Prior to the pandemic, I used to check in with my students via phone call and email. Now, due to COVID-19, I prioritize Zoom calls so my students can safely interact with someone outside of their bubble. These meetings help my students receive real-time answers to their questions and also provides them an outlet to express how they are feeling. Outside of my students, my colleagues and I have weekly Zoom meetings which help us to sync our priorities and discuss issues that need solving. While my colleagues and I don't need to have these meetings weekly, we've found that these video meetings keep communication lines open, fosters social interaction, and keeps us engaged.

Establish Expectations. Working from home has many more distractions than the average workplace so that is why it is important to establish expectations. This tip is in tandem with establishing a routine. Not only should you be clear about what your working hours should be, but you should also establish expectations about your work too. If your office utilizes Google Calendar, block off times on the calendar that you need for deep working. For my students, I make sure to reiterate that even though a pandemic is occurring, I expect them to follow the syllabus, engage in meaningful discussions, and turn in their work in a timely fashion. Establishing these clear expectations helps not only ensure successful classroom instruction but also allows the student to succeed too and helps the student learn and apply the information, too.

Watch your tone and body language. While we may not realize it, our tone and body language are more important than our actual spoken word. There is a pervasive belief that 55% of our communication is through body language, 38% is the tone of voice, and 7% is actual words spoken.[10] When we no longer can communicate in person, our written words become even more important and carry more weight. Before sending an email, reread it several times to make sure your point is coming across well and your thoughts are legible. Avoid using vague words like "it" "that" "them" and try to be as concise as possible. When on a video call, make sure you appear alert and use nonverbal cues (like nodding your head) and verbal cues (your voice) to confirm your understanding.

BE KIND TO YOURSELF

As offices closed around the country due to COVID-19, millions of Americans are now working remotely and learning to navigate this "new normal." Prior to the pandemic, remote work may have been a welcomed perk to many employees but now, remote work has made many employees stressed, overwhelmed, and lonely. Even as an 11-year veteran of remote work, I have also struggled with feelings of isolation and worried about the unknown.

It is important to acknowledge these feelings and accept them, no matter how painful they are. Give yourself permission to take breaks when you feel your concentration start to lag. Although I schedule breaks during my workday, there are some days where I need to take a few more nonscheduled breaks. I will take a break from my computer and walk around my house just to refocus my mind and get a change of scenery.

Working remotely can be a struggle for even the most experienced veteran of remote work. Being physically removed from coworkers and the office environment is a hurdle that can take a toll on your focus, as well as your productivity at times. While some days seem may feel like everything is running smoothly, others may have more of a start/stop type feeling to them. What is important is to not let these variances weigh too heavily on your mind.

Remote Learning in Perilous Times

When I attended college in the 1980s, remote learning was not even a concept. After college, I proceeded to work in corporate America and raise a family. In 2001, I obtained my MBA from Davenport University in strategic management and leadership. At that point, I decided to go for my PhD but was unsure of what avenue to take. I could have taken traditional ground classes, but I also needed to work to support my family. I eventually discovered that Capella University—a Minneapolis based school—was offering an online PhD program. This program would allow me not only to work but to also take classes too. I leapt at the opportunity.

In the early to mid-2000s, online instruction was very different than it is today, and I would argue that it was much more challenging and complicated. While instructors were responsive, there would be a 12- to 24-hour delay in responses. Learning the course material was on the student and it was up to us to teach ourselves the course material and do our own research to validate what we were learning. Instead of video conferencing, we were required to fly to the school and attend colloquial four times a year. Colloquial was an opportunity to meet your professors face to face, network with your peers, and attend weekend seminars and lectures. Even back then, online learning was a choice and only restricted to so many students at a time.

Enter COVID-19, a virus that has forced the entire world to hunker down in our homes for the foreseeable future. Universities and colleges that mostly dealt with traditional ground classes had to scramble to accommodate a complete shift to online learning by shifting as many courses as possible to online and hoping that the technological platforms could handle the high usage levels. For universities and colleges that mostly dealt with online instruction—like Sullivan University—the shift to fully online learning was more seamless. I firmly believe that Sullivan's success in moving all classes online was due to Sullivan's determined push to have faculty trained in online instruction and that Sullivan invested in quality technological platforms that could handle high usage levels.

In order for students to receive the best education possible during these trying times, I believe that online synchronous learning should be emphasized. Synchronous learning is when the instructor and the student are in the same place, at the same time for live instruction.[11] This is the typical collegiate learning method. The student attends class and listens to an instructor lecture. The student is able to ask questions and receive an answer immediately. Asynchronous learning allows the student to learn at their own pace by engaging with the course material at different times and places than the instruction actually took place.[12] This is typically seen in traditional online learning. The student is able to log in to their school's technological platform and learn the course material on their own time.

For students who actively choose online learning, asynchronous instruction works well because the students already know the expectations of online instruction and can engage in the course at their own direction. For students who prefer in-person instruction, asynchronous instruction may be more difficult for them as they may not believe they are receiving the same type of education they would have received if they were synchronously learning.

While I believe that synchronous learning should be emphasized during perilous times, I also recognize that asynchronous learning has its benefits too. Synchronous online learning is possible by utilizing videoconferencing platforms. For example, I will post an announcement in the course that I will be recording a live lecture and any student is welcome to join. The students that are able to join can actively participate in the lecture and I have the ability to clarify any misconceptions of the material before they take root in the student's mind. However, I am cognizant that not all students are able to make it to live lectures so I ensure that all lectures are recorded so all my students can benefit from the material and can then call me or schedule a Zoom call to discuss any questions they may have.

COVID-19's effects and ramifications will be far-reaching and will be studied even after the pandemic is over. Until we are able to firmly get a grip on this virus we will have to adjust to our "new normal," which includes remote working and remote learning. For remote working, it is important for employees to keep their work and home lives separate in order to keep the lines between the work environment and home environment clear, to create a routine as if you are going into the office in order to put yourself in the correct headspace to work, to establish or join a community in order to stave off loneliness and to be part of a work culture, utilize technology and communication to maximize your remote work experience, and to be kind to yourself. For remote learning, a mixture of synchronous learning and asynchronous learning is key to maximizing learning.

NOTES

1. https://wwwnc.cdc.gov/eid/article/26/6/20-0516_article
2. https://covid.cdc.gov/covid-data-tracker/#datatracker-home (as of the writing of this chapter, the current United States death toll is 510,577)
3. https://www.michigan.gov/whitmer/0,9309,7-387-90499_90705-524032--,00.html (this Executive Order was rescinded by Executive Order 2020-65)
4. https://www.fox2detroit.com/news/governors-goal-of-returning-michigan-students-to-in-person-learning-is-today (this article found that certain school districts, like the Detroit Public Schools, had not released re-opening plans but were expected to re-open their doors sometime in March 2021).
5. https://www.courier-journal.com/story/news/education/2020/03/11/how-kentucky-colleges-universities-responding-coronavirus-outbreak/5020013002/
6. https://www.prweb.com/releases/sullivan_university_launching_online_summer_quarter_june_29/prweb17160480.htm
7. https://www.forbes.com/sites/ashleystahl/2020/04/06/5-habits-for-a-morning-routine-if-you-work-from-home/?sh=6846802ae424
8. https://www.forbes.com/sites/benjaminlaker/2020/08/24/working-from-home-is-disliked-by-and-bad-for-most-employees/?sh=12b6a98e6734
9. https://www.forbes.com/sites/benjaminlaker/2020/08/24/working-from-home-is-disliked-by-and-bad-for-most-employees/?sh=12b6a98e6734 (Prior to the pandemic, 62% of surveyed employees reported they had positive mental health)
10. https://www.psychologytoday.com/us/blog/beyond-words/201109/is-nonverbal-communication-numbers-game (These percentages do not apply to every situation and should not be used to try and analyze every situation)
11. https://www.brynmawr.edu/blendedlearning/asynchronous-vs-synchronous-learning-quick-overview
12. https://www.brynmawr.edu/blendedlearning/asynchronous-vs-synchronous-learning-quick-overview

CHAPTER 17

ACADEMIC CHALLENGES OF VIRTUAL CLASSES DURING THE PANDEMIC

An Elementary ESL Teacher's Perspective

Joanne Rodriguez Addarich

INTRODUCTION

The COVID-19 pandemic has undoubtedly forced a transformation of societal routines. The world's economies, the healthcare sector, education, sports and entertainment have all suffered a long lasting impact. It is also likely that human behavior has undergone significant change. One particular area that was severely disrupted is schooling. This chapter focuses on the pandemic effects within the elementary educational system. The field of education is a vital area given its ultimate goal of educating our younger population who stand to become the future leaders of our society. The impact of the pandemic on elementary school children can be best captured by a couple of statistics. Li and Lalani (2020) suggested that over 1.2 billion children worldwide were taken out of the classrooms when the pandemic began in early 2020. In addition, the pandemic has brought about the return of children up to 11 years of age to daycare.

Back to a New Normal: In Search of Stability in an Era of Pandemic Disruption—Insight From Practitioners and Academics, pp. 241–249

These statistics illustrate the magnitude of disruption caused to young students, along with their parents and teachers.

The next few pages of this article succinctly capture the perspectives of a few elementary teachers concerning the effects of the pandemic, remote learning and related classroom modifications that followed, as well as their implications for the future. The small sample of teachers from elementary public schools in Kentucky and New York included an English as a secondary language (ESL) elementary teacher, a kindergarten teacher, a teacher's assistant, and a social studies/special education elementary teacher. The focus is on their experiences with virtual classes during the pandemic.

A NEW COURSE IN TEACHING/LEARNING PROCESSES

Teachers found themselves amidst a sudden and a radical disruption that took place, allowing for a very short time frame to prepare and execute classroom tasks and activities using a virtual platform. Changes were to be made not only in terms of academics and curriculum, but also as to how to engage the students and provide an effective teaching/learning experience. These adjustments required additional technological training in order to be successful with the new modality of virtual classes. The teachers, the students, and the parents received new instructions on how to use technological devices and the applications for the virtual classes that were going to be taking place.

This instructional transformation challenged all school stakeholders and especially the youngest students and oldest caretakers. The fast pace with which all these modifications to the traditional teaching/learning model occurred caused teachers to become physically and emotionally stressed. Although processes and procedures were reinvented by the tail of the school year, new arrangements took place amidst uncertain, frightening, and stressful times triggered by the horrific Corona virus. Nonetheless, *the job needed to get done.*

Many labels have been given to programs' implementation within the school system and to the necessary adjustments made. Labeling in this particular case was challenging due to the unique and unusual manner in which these adaptations were established. Fisher et al. (2021) explain in their book *The Distance Learning Playbook* that teaching during 2020 was not to be considered distance learning or homeschooling, but that it was indeed crisis teaching. A distinction among the terms is necessary in order to understand the importance of self-care in the aftermath of the changes made in the elementary education system during the 2020–2021 period.

THE IMPORTANCE OF SELF-CARE

Self-care has been a very important teaching quality worthy of observation during the COVID-19 era. School social workers and family resource specialists were assigned the responsibility of providing both teachers and students with tools to cope with this matter. Self-care became a priority so as to minimize the level of anxiety that a sudden and unexpected change in the middle of the school year might cause. Teachers, students, and caretakers all faced instances in which circumstances required adapting to new challenges and at the same time remain strong and resilient.

Great importance was given to self-care as a critical practice and a new norm. Consider that Fisher et al. (2021) stressed the role of self-care. They contend that a teacher cannot prepare for crisis teaching without considering her/his own state of health and most importantly one's emotional state. They also state that, though teachers are prepared for and are trained to work in an environment full of children with smiling and welcoming faces, the pandemic disrupted this historical pattern. This disruption created a new reality completely different from what a teacher had come to expect and was prepared for.

And again, one should recall that normal classes transitioned into this new crisis modality in the middle of the school year. And for that reason, teachers needed to prepare themselves for crisis teaching while operating in good physical and emotional health. It is important to note that, during times of crisis, individuals can experience a resurfacing of past traumatic episodes which might lead to difficulties managing the present experience. Students' state of mind and emotional health were equally, if not even more important. In an effort to make the transition easier for the students, engagement acquired a new definition during the pandemic.

ENGAGING TO LEARN AND LEARNING TO ENGAGE

Once virtual classes began, additional concerns and situations arose given the existence of synchronous and asynchronous classes. Initially, the main concern was how often students logged in to synchronous classes and with what regularity in order to complete asynchronous assignments. For both teachers and students, acquiring new technological skills were critical for successful teaching of synchronous classes and for preparing successful asynchronous classes. Districts and teachers took quick actions to deliver computers to the students and provide them access to the internet. Once these logistics were achieved, the next goal was to develop instructional content and relevant class materials to ensure sound student engagement.

Materials developed included choice boards for the first few weeks which provided educators with time to train on how to use different technological tools in their classes. Several hours of training were needed to learn how to properly use the tools and incorporate them into the classroom. By and large, this effort was positively welcomed by most educators; the few who did not eventually were compelled to come around to acceptance. Class engagement is key in order to be successful in the learning/teaching process. Different Google and Microsoft tools became popular and essential during the first part of the pandemic. Companies that provide technological resources for teaching improved their products and created new products. Educational technology has become a great teaching ally, and it is clearly here to stay.

The modality of student engagement has always been an area of concern in the teaching process, and institutions that had adopted the modality prepandemic continued to reflect upon it as they implemented their virtual classes. Engagement methods and strategies vary between synchronous and asynchronous classes, according to the learning style of students. A study of students' preferences regarding synchronous and asynchronous classes yielded a few important findings. Misbah et al. (2017) assessed students' preferences across the two modalities, and reported that the presence of a moderator in synchronous classes is of high importance and makes a difference as to the level of class engagement.

An additional factor that is present in synchronous classes is the sense of self-contribution; this factor has emerged as another meaningful variable for students (Misbah et al., 2017, p. 185). The authors stressed the importance of a greater sense of assignment completion, along with the higher rate of focusing during synchronous classes. Some students preferred asynchronous classes due to the time related flexibility provided by this type of class (p. 186). The authors emphasized the importance of considering the physical, social, emotional, and psychological state of the students while planning both synchronous and asynchronous classes as such states contribute to the level of student engagement.

It is of major significance that the pandemic did not provide sufficient lead time for planning and that virtual learning was implemented with very little experience in elementary and secondary level schools. These schools found themselves at a disadvantage compared with institutions of higher learning who have been offering remote learning platforms for years. This fact burdened the virtual delivery in schools to an even greater extent. It is also important to note that most school systems in the United States are still learning how to make maximum use of these virtual platforms. Remote learning continues to be re-evaluated and modified, and it is likely to continue to evolve and develop in the face of future pandemics that are likely to occur.

TEACHERS' OPINIONS ABOUT THE IMPACT OF THE PANDEMIC IN THEIR CLASSROOMS

The following are informal brief interviews the author conducted with fellow teachers. Obviously, this collection of teachers' opinions is designed only to illustrate teachers experiences during a chaotic period of time. It is inevitable that teachers talk about the impact of the pandemic on students in their classrooms. The author had a conversation with a teacher and her assistant from the same public school district in the state of Kentucky. They are very experienced and skilled elementary teachers; the author teaches ESL, and her peer teaches kindergarten. A second conversation was held with a social studies/special education elementary teacher from a public school district in New York. Lastly, the author reflects on her own teaching experience during the pandemic.

Ms. P.M. (Kindergarten Teacher From a Kentucky Public Elementary School)

1. What kind of impact has the pandemic had on your relationship with your students?

> The impact has been severe on a daily emotional side. I do not have the same emotional relationship with students because the opportunity to interact in the classroom has been eliminated due to the pandemic. Without in-Person interactions, I am unable to build a trusting relationship that comes from meeting students' daily school needs. These needs vary from opening lunch packages to applying a band-aid in order to calm tears from a scraped knee.

2. Have you seen a difference in academic achievement and performance among your students receiving virtual classes as opposed to in-person classes?

> Academic achievement and performance are dismal in a virtual class, and stand in contrast to the higher level achieved with in-person classes. Given the percentage of material taught in the virtual format based on state standards, only 10%–20% of completion in school curriculum has been achieved."

3. As a teacher, what is your general opinion concerning virtual classes?

   I absolutely loved teaching virtual! I would like to continue developing a virtual curriculum for elementary students.

4. Describe your experience with synchronous and asynchronous classes in terms of students' participation and engagement.

   My experience is teaching synchronous with Google Meets and asynchronous with Google Classroom has been very positive. I found there is a wide range of learning options for students based on personal preference, time and familial situations.

5. Have communication with your students' parents been different while using virtual classes modality compared to in-person modality? Please explain your answer.

   Communication has been very productive compared to in-person. I have 3 scheduled daily opportunities to be in touch with parents, guardians and older siblings—these include Google Meet synchronous twice a day and an office hour conducted through both synchronous and asynchronous modalities. Because I teach elementary students, there is generally an adult or older sibling available at all times.

Ms. M.A.H. (Kindergarten Teacher's Assistant From a Kentucky Public Elementary School)

1. How would you describe your experience with virtual classes?

   I have enjoyed learning the tools that exist for meeting virtually. I found the kids needed extra support to keep them engaged during class.

2. What is your general opinion concerning virtual classes? Pros:

   Teaching has become more intense in order to meet requirements of instructional time.

   Behavioral issues have been minimized with synchronous classes versus in-person.

   I enjoy virtual classes because it facilitates working with small groups and the students have equal accessibility to resources because they are virtual.

I think that technology has improved classes tremendously and it should be incorporated during in-person classes. School districts need to invest in updated technology to improve the curriculum.

Cons:

I think that kids may not acquire full learning during virtual classes due to under-utilization of all five senses. For that reason, I believe in-person classes are more productive.

Children's interaction with their peers is pretty much non-existent in virtual classes. They often do not know each other's names. Social skills in my opinion start at a young age and are critical for future success.

I think in person classes are safer, richer in content and experience, and also in terms of overall efficiency.

Mr. M.F. (Social Studies/Special Education Teacher From a New York Public Elementary School)

1. How would you describe your experience with virtual classes during the pandemic?

Due to virtual classes, some parents have complained about their children not learning, and having less structure and interaction with their friends. If teachers are technologically savvy, the learning process is much easier. As a teacher I believe nothing replaces in-person instruction and being able to work collectively in groups and most importantly providing individualized instruction. Special education students have different learning styles and needs, and their service providers (speech, occupational, and physical therapy, etc.) are guided by an [Individual Education Plan]. These students require a hands-on teaching and learning environment. I believe that behavioral, emotional, and learning disabilities have to be addressed in person.

Ms. J.R (ESL Teacher at a Public Elementary School in Kentucky)

As an ESL teacher, my charge is to prepare new students in the public school system, who have English limitations by virtue of it not being their first language. I must meet their individual language needs and assist with cultural adaptation as well. Being an immigrant myself, I can strongly relate to my students. The pandemic has presented challenges for everyone. However, my students face the additional challenge of having family members and relatives who themselves have English language limitations. These conditions can

> present themselves as both academic and emotional barriers to students during these difficult pandemic times.
>
> Another requirement of my job is communicating with parents; The goal is to keep them informed about their child's progress but also to keep them informed about school policies and procedures along with district services. Some parents lost their jobs during the pandemic. Others struggled to balance work and helping their children with synchronous and asynchronous classes. I have to admit I had more opportunities to see my students during virtual classes.
>
> I taught synchronous classes because I prefer to see my students live. Seeing students in small groups helps me maintain a good working relationship with them. Being now on a hybrid schedule, I still use synchronous classes for virtual student instruction as well as parental meetings. The hybrid method prevents me from seeing my students as much as I would like due to children attending school only 2 days a week. Prior to the pandemic I planned my schedule according to student priority needs, and toward that end, students that most needed my attention would gain more class hours during the week.
>
> In my opinion nothing substitutes for personal interaction between teacher/student and student/student. Children also learn by doing and through hands on application, and, most importantly, they learn from each other.

Teachers who shared their opinions, agreed that engagement and relationships with their students are the most important instructional features during the COVID-19 pandemic era. Teachers likewise share a genuine, over-riding concern for their students wellbeing, even elevating this factor above their own needs. Given that teachers are often not considering their own self-care, it is therefore understandable why administrators and educational experts emphasize the need to place a high priority on teachers' self-care.

CONCLUSION

Teacher-student relationships have been the most critical aspect of virtual classes and the one aspect teachers are most concerned about. Relationships with students feature prominently in educational settings, and particularly in the classroom. The teacher is a moderator and an inspirer, a guide and a consoler in their classroom. Therefore, the relationship between teacher and student is one that should not be taken lightly. Fisher et al. (2021) argue that one common denominator among teachers, when asked about the key aspect that matter the most in the learning process, is the relationship with the students (p. 47). Creating a relationship with the students occurs in the classroom at all times. A teacher observes the students' nonverbal communication, as well as listen to the students' feedback, comments, and ideas. The classroom provides a perfect setting for fostering healthy and productive interaction, and for providing positive feedback to students. This critical aspect, if not eliminated altogether, has been reduced during the pandemic and the imposed virtual environment that has been created.

It has been proven during the pandemic that humans certainly are resilient beings; teachers are not an exception. Educators have been giving their very best in making the teaching-learning process possible despite the challenging times. It is uncertain still what educational gaps have been widened, and what deficits in learning have been created during and post pandemic. However, there is no question that technology is here to stay, and that when properly used, it can be a great ally.

AUTHOR'S NOTE

Special thanks to the fellow teachers that collaborated with their opinions about virtual classes.

REFERENCES

Fisher, D., Frey, N., & Hattie, J.(2021). *The distance learning playbook teaching for engagement & impact in any setting*. Corwin.

Lalani, F., & Li, C. (2020, April 29). The COVID-19 pandemic has changed education forever. This is how. *World Economic Forum*. https://www.weforum.org/agenda/2020/04/coronavirus-education-global-covid19-online-digital-learning

Misbah, M., Ghulam, F., Abid, H., & Ayesha, S. (2017). E-learning: Students' perspectives about asynchronous and synchronous resources at higher education level. *Bulletin of Education and Research*, 183–195.

CHAPTER 18

RESETTING THE NORM

Leveraging the Pandemics to Increase Equity in Education

J. Claudette Howard

INTRODUCTION

Thursday evening, March 12, 2020, the world stopped. This unforgettable day marks the moment when the state of Kentucky's largest public school district sent an email to thousands of employees and the families of over 90,000 students stating that all schools would be closed for the next few weeks due to health concerns around COVID-19. According to that infamous email, students were to return to their regular school schedule on April 6, 2020, following a 2-week break because of concerns about the spread of COVID-19 and 1 week for their previously planned spring break. This email and decision triggered many thoughts and multiple perspectives but one thing that no one imagined at that time, was that teachers, staff, and administrators would not reenter school buildings with students again until March 17, 2021.

Corona virus disease 19 (COVID-19) is an infectious respiratory illness that is spread through fluids from the mouths and noses of infected people (World Health Organization, 2021). Since its discovery in December

Back to a New Normal: In Search of Stability in an Era of Pandemic Disruption—Insight From Practitioners and Academics, pp. 251–264

2019 there have been close to 169 million reported cases of COVID-19 and 3.51 million deaths worldwide, over 33 million reported cases and 590,000 deaths nationwide, and 459,000 cases reported in Kentucky with nearly 7,000 dead (*The New York Times*, 2020). As this disease spread across the globe, it triggered panic and preparation worldwide. One of the first places that it affected in the US was public schools. In early 2020, there were reports of cases in various countries, but it was not until mid-February when the American Federation of Teachers called for guidance around handling the disease, that district and school administrators really began to take notice (*Education Week*, 2020).

It was shortly after this that the Centers for Disease Control and Prevention warned schools and families that closures were imminent but still, these adjustments were at the behest of individual schools/districts. Beginning in late February, some schools and districts chose to do short term closures to address isolated infections and to contemplate the impact of having to close longer term. Conversations were had, think pieces were written, but on March 11, 2020, when COVID-19 was declared a pandemic (a disease that has risen to prevalence across the world), education leadership had no choice but to close schools to in-person learning.

To say that the pandemic mandated major shifts to teaching methods would be an understatement. While educators left school buildings one spring and did not physically return until a year later, they still had to continue to teach children how to read, write, do math, and to be caring empathetic people, only virtually instead of in-person. The moral imperative to educate our youth is not a short order in a "normal" school setting but to quote our superintendent and a member of the engineering team in Apollo 13, when the pandemic forced us to move school to the internet, we had to, "put a square peg in a round hole ... rapidly." Now educators are not strangers to flexibility and changing plans on the fly so of course, they made arrangements. Schools and districts who already had models of nontraditional instruction (NTI) for severe weather or other acts of God changed course to implement these programs for a longer term. Districts who did not already have a standing system for online instruction quickly put plans together and submitted them to the state for approval. Schools lined up to empty their inventory of personal computers to ensure that each student had a device and organized the purchase of hotspots to ensure that students who were at high risk of learning loss had access to a reliable internet connection.

Families also began to adjust. Homeschooling schedules and "classroom" setups started popping up on social media. Families sat down together each evening to watch their governor's daily coronavirus briefing. Even something as unique as "drive by" parties became the norm. It was not surprising to be sitting quietly in your home in the evening only to be drawn to the window by people honking their horns and shouting from brightly decorated vehicles heralding the birthday, anniversary, graduation, etcetera of whoever on whatever day.

Masks gradually turned from an oddity to an accessory, and there were few neighborhoods where you could walk more than a few feet without stepping on a freshly designed chalk drawings. If we did not know any better, we might have thought that people were living the dream, minimizing, getting back to the basics, spending time with family, considering work life balance and whatever other attractive way we decide to describe being stuck at home in the middle of a global crisis. Unfortunately, this surface level calm was not the whole story.

With school buildings closed and "school" online, parents and guardians were at a loss for what to do with their children. Although many businesses also switched to virtual platforms, there were many other places of business that remained open. This left parents with a conundrum, go to work and leave their children unattended or stay home and possibly lose their job. Even those who were working from home struggled to balance completing their daily work and caring for their children at the same time. Not only that, teachers and administrators were at home dealing with the same issues while simultaneously trying to educate their students.

By April 2020, only a month after businesses and schools began closing their doors to in-person traffic there were already nearly 400,000 unemployment applications in Kentucky alone; nearly 20% of the state's workforce (Tobin, 2020). By May, that number was still climbing and was 938 percent higher than the number of unemployment claims from May of the previous year (Latek, 2020). While these numbers are dire, they do not even begin to tell the full story of the destruction wrought by the COVID-19 pandemic.

To fully address the devastating impact of this pandemic, we must acknowledge the physical toll that it placed on Kentuckians, Americans, and humans worldwide; as well as the financial, social, emotional, mental health, and academic challenges that resulted from and were magnified by loss, change in lifestyle, and the myriad of other problems. All of these challenges inevitably affected the quality of education that teachers were able to give and that students are able to receive, which begs the question, "How has the COVID-19 pandemic impacted educators' ability to provide equitable access to a free and appropriate education for every child?" Before we begin attempting to answer this question, however, it is also important to note that even prior to the pandemic, schools were struggling to reliably provide effective education for all students (Redding & Nguyen, 2020).

For decades, the education community in our nation has been criticized for its failure to consistently produce proficient outcomes in students; especially students from diverse backgrounds, students with special needs, and students who are living in poverty (Borman, 2005; Borman et al., 2003; Plunkett, 1985; Puma & Drury, 2000). As a principal of an accelerated improvement school, or more commonly, a "turnaround" school, this fact is never too far from my mind. This is why I cannot possibly provide my practitioner perspective on the impact of the COVID-19 pandemic on K–12 education without also asking "How do we mitigate the effects of this pandemic in a system where the students most affected were already experiencing disproportionate negative effects from an inherently racist educational system?"

In addition to dealing with the medical (physical and mental health), social, emotional, academic, and financial consequences of the COVID-19 pandemic, over the past year, educators in America have also been embroiled in another pandemic; that system racism and its effect on public schooling. In this chapter, racism is defined as, "a system of privilege and oppression, a network of traditions, legitimating standards, material and institutional arrangements, and ideological apparatuses that, together, serve to perpetuate hierarchical social relations based on race" (Thompson, 1997, p. 9). More simply, racism is a system of oppression that is designed to disenfranchise some groups and benefit another. In the United States, norms are based on whiteness and in order for this construct to persist, it is necessary for non-Whiteness and most notably Blackness to be considered beneath and problematic to whiteness (Feagin, 2013; Holst, 2020; Inoue, 2017; Thompson, 1997). This is true in both the structure of this nation and in the systems designed by the leadership that maintains this structure. This includes our public education system.

The fact that systemic racism is inseparable from our nation's education system is not news. Enslaved Africans were completely denied access to education but even when slavery "ended" *Plessy v. Ferguson* (1896) ensured that Black people continued to have limited access (Parkerson & Parkerson, 2014). And even in the years after *Brown v. Board of Education* (1955) "desegregated" schools, it still took 34 years before even 40% of Black students attended integrated primarily white schools. Only 14 years ago the Supreme Court ruled that using race as the primary factor for student assignment in Jefferson County Public Schools was unconstitutional (Egelko, 2007; Totenberg & Kaufman, 2007). But access to school choice is only the tip of the injustice iceberg. Black students also continue to receive harsh discipline (suspension, arrest, and expulsion) more frequently than their white counterparts (Riddle & Sinclair, 2019) as well as achieve at lower levels than white students regardless of the Black students' socioeconomic status (Lubienski, 2002). As disturbing as these persistent inequities are, they are definitely not new information. How then, is it possible, that educators can plan to effectively address the "COVID slide" and not actively engage in antiracist action? It is impossible to ignore this other, older and more insidious pandemic and hope to be effective in accelerating students beyond the compounded damage from the new one.

What follows is a description of my experience as a school leader finishing a year and beginning another one in virtual learning. I will end by summarizing lessons I learned and how I plan to use them as leverage to accelerate students beyond the achievement gaps, opportunity gaps, and belief gaps that existed before COVID-19.

NAVIGATING THE TRANSITION TO ONLINE LEARNING

February 2020 was a rough month at the elementary school where I served as assistant principal. Flu A, flue B, strep throat, and pneumonia had decimated both student and teacher attendance, so as March began, we were excited to finally get back to business as usual. We were aware of the news about COVID-19, but when compared to what we'd experienced during flu season, classrooms with as few as six students in them, we did not expect much different from this new virus. As the days passed however, and reports of the "novel coronavirus" became more and more frequent, we began to see the writing on the wall. We passed out Clorox wipes and hand sanitizer, things that had previously been off limits for classrooms, and started to incorporate lessons and procedures for cleaning and handwashing into our established routines. It was at this point that the emails started to change in tone.

The first thing that clued us in to a major change was when we were told that parents reporting "concerns" about the spread of the coronavirus was an acceptable excuse for students missing school. The next red flag was when we started to receive emails about the curriculum development department designing activities for students to do independently in the event that we had to be home for an extended period, which at the time we all believed, if it happened, would only be a few weeks to get quarantines out of the way around spring break.

At our school, we also began organizing schoolwork and activities that we could send home with students if we had to stop coming to school. The way that we designed instruction at our school, was slightly different from the norm, so we wanted to put our own spin on things to ensure that students could continue to move in the right direction. We also began reaching out to families to determine whether or not students had technology at home. Every student at our school had a Chromebook, but at that time, these devices remained at school and did not travel back and forth with students.

As the days progressed and it became more and more clear that school buildings would be closing and that very few students had reliable access to technology at home, some administrators received notification that we would have to turn over our devices to disperse to students throughout the district. This was shocking news. As a Title I school, we knew that most of our students did not have technology at home and we wanted to send them home with the devices that we had purchased for them. Rather than doing this, however, the district had decided to collect as many devices as they could and then design a system to distribute them. This system did not exist on the day that schools closed to in-person school. All we knew, was that we should remove the devices from their carts and leave them in an easily accessible area for district staff to collect.

Shortly after students were sent home, administrators and other school staff, with the exception of housekeeping were also told to leave school buildings. We spent the next several weeks at our homes trying to contact students, check on their well-being, and determine which students had devices and who did not. By this time, the district had decided to send the devices that they had collected through mail to students who qualified for free/reduced lunch, students who had Individual Education Plans, and students who were learning English. At this time, the process was time consuming and complicated and so some students did not receive devices until shortly before the end of the school year or at all. Fortunately, the district also worked to create a system to distribute paper packets to students who did not have access to a device, internet services, or who could not access the free trials that some service providers were offering. Last, the district designated certain schools as sites where children could go to pick up food for breakfast and lunch.

While the district and school staff were working together to get students outfitted with technology, paper packets, and food, teachers and administrators were designing plans to teach students online using a variety of approved platforms. The state department of education created guidelines for tracking online participation as well as expectations that limited the amount of work assigned and the number of hours students were required to be in front of a screen. This process of lesson design was less difficult for our school because of our process for collaborative planning. Prior to the beginning of the fourth instructional cycle, we had already outlined the objectives for the final unit, so we only had to plan lessons and assignments that aligned with these units.

This, however, was not the norm. Most schools spent the brief period between the announcement of school closures and the beginning of NTI scrambling to pull together a smattering of district created curriculum and online resources, many of which they did not have time to vet. Also, there was an enormous amount of time and energy being spent just locating students and trying maintain an open line of communication with families. Because of this unique situation, during NTI, student attendance was more fluid, and schools were advised to mark participation instead of daily attendance. This meant that any contact, including a call or text with a parent, a student logging in to an online platform, a picture sent to a teacher's email, or logging into an online meeting counted as a "contact." The state did not want families to be "punished" if they had limited access to technology, so the rules around truancy were softened during this time. If students were completing work or if their parents continued to communicate with the teacher, students could be given credit for participation equivalent to the amount of work completed or the number of contacts made (Kentucky Department of Education, 2020).

In terms of teacher attendance, our district administration worked with the teacher's union to agree upon an altered schedule for them as well. Just like our students' families, classroom teachers and school staff were now working from home and responsible for their own children in addition to the students in their classes. In an effort to show flexibility and support, the collaborative committee comprised of school and district administrators and representatives from the teachers' union developed a daily work schedule for teachers that included approximately three and a half hours for teaching and three and a half hours for planning. There was a "suggested" daily schedule that broke the planning time down but nothing that outlined the teaching time. It is my belief, as an educator and as a parent, that this lack of clarity on what constituted, "teaching" time is where the infamous "COVID-19" slide began.

Imagine that education was doing your hair in the morning. If teaching were a hair tie, then online instruction was the third twist. You know, when you are trying to get that high ponytail just right and you pull the elastic to the farthest it can go to get that last twist in and the whole thing just snaps? Yes, that is what happened last spring. Now, I am not arguing that NTI broke teaching, what I want to illustrate is that when school went to the virtual platform en masse, the tenuous fidelity of what constituted teaching collapsed. In a time when concerns about safety and access to resources made learning more difficult than it has ever been, the idea of what qualified as effective instruction became more abstract and, in many cases, the role of the teacher was greatly diminished.

Many schools responded to the relaxed expectations around teaching by designing plans that relied heavily on asynchronous instruction. This ranged from schools offering only four days of live teaching to schools only offering students one short meeting with their teacher each week. During the year that our district was all digital, I transitioned from being an assistant principal at one school, to the principal of another. There were innumerable differences between my former school and my current one when I arrived, but the one difference that is most relevant to this chapter is the fact that the school I came from offered live instruction to students five days a week and my new school had operated on the other end of the spectrum to close out the previous school year.

This was one of the first things that I addressed when I arrived in July of 2020 but that does not change the fact that the students at my current school, an accelerated improvement school, one that is designated as scoring in the bottom five percent of schools in the state, finished the 2020–2021 school year without each student receiving the maximum amount of synchronous instruction allowed. I am not highlighting this difference to criticize or downplay the work that occurred before my tenure. I am only using it as an example from my personal experience to illustrate the variability of digital learning between two schools in the same district. The fact that two schools, not even six miles apart, one, having only just exited the bottom five percent and the other getting its third principal in 3 years could have such incredibly different perspectives on what online learning looks like is concerning. It is also a microcosm of the lack of consistency in education that was happening across the nation during the apex of the COVID-19 pandemic.

While digital learning in a pandemic is only a recently burgeoning area of research, there is a body of literature around best practices in digital learning. In response to the COVID-19 pandemic, the Education Endowment Foundation (2020) tapped into this data and completed a rapid evidence assessment of remote learning. This meta-analysis included 60 studies (distilled from over 3,500 studies) and found no clear difference between synchronous and asynchronous instruction in terms of learning and that the teaching quality was more important than the lesson delivery. We must bear in mind, however, that this study is limited by the fact that the literature analyzed was mainly focused on postsecondary education. The authors explicitly stated that before applying any of their conclusions to school-aged children, careful consideration was needed.

They also highlighted the importance of providing access to technology to all students, specifically those from marginalized communities and to peer interaction as a factor to improve engagement and student outcomes during online learning (Education Endowment Foundation, 2020). In addition, they provided the caveat that school leaders and teachers must use their "professional judgment" prior to repurposing technology that was meant to be used by students *in school* and applying it to remote learning. So, even with remote learning, what matters most in student outcomes is teacher effectiveness, teacher efficacy, student engagement, and equity of access; the same things that improve student outcomes in in-person school (Hattie & Zierer, 2018). How unfortunate then that many students spent a large part of their time using online programs rather than hearing from their teacher.

The importance of teachers to student learning is an undisputed fact (Blasé & Blasé, 1999; Dwyer, 1985; Heck & Hallinger, 1999; Leithwood & Duke, 1999; Leithwood et al., 2008; New Leaders for New Schools, 2009; Portin et al., 2009; Smith & Andrews, 1989) and it is why one of my first orders of business when I became principal in July 2020, was to design an NTI plan that made sure that every student at our school saw a teacher each day and that each teacher was provided with professional development that ensured that they grew in effectiveness and efficacy. The driving goal for our school turnaround is to make sure that each student has access to rigorous, engaging, standards-based learning experiences that cater to his or her culture. We are also compelled to provide teachers with professional development and monitoring that supports them in being able to reliably provide these types of experiences to students.

These are the improvement priorities from our state department of education and if we do not progress toward proficiency in these areas, I, as the principal am in danger of losing my job. Ultimately, success in turnaround, will be measured using the results of the state assessment and not merely be measured by looking at our school as a whole, but also looking at each subgroup of students including Black students, Hispanic students, students who qualify for free and reduced Lunch, and students who qualify for Individual Education Plans or in the ESL program. These, "achievement gaps" existed before COVID-19 and were created and continue to exist because of systemic racism that exists in this country (Redding & Nguyen, 2020). This is why it is impossible to discuss a remedy for the COVID-19 slide without talking about the persistent injustice perpetrated by the public school systems in our nation. Because, while many students need a lifeboat to recover from the COVID-19 school closures, there were students who were already drowning who now need a submarine.

BRIDGING THE GAPS

Prior to the COVID-19 pandemic there were schools and districts receiving federal funds who were struggling to accelerate diverse groups of students to proficiency while at the same time employing methods that further increased the divide. The last time students in Kentucky took the state assessment for accountability, it was in spring of 2019 and there were dozens of schools, in my district alone, who did not meet their goals for student growth or proficiency. It is now 2 years later, and we are still responsible for closing these gaps, only now, they are wider and deeper, and the target is still moving. So, as a principal, what do you do when you thought you were swimming the English Channel but instead you are navigating the Marianas Trench? The answer is you do whatever is necessary.

What follows are lessons I learned during the COVID-19 school closures that have helped me grow in my first year as a turnaround principal.

1. **Prioritize teacher efficacy.** One of the blessings of the pandemic has been the ability to spend more time with teachers. Collective teacher efficacy is the highest yield instructional strategy for student acceleration (Hattie & Zierer, 2018). Having the opportunity this year, as a new principal, to meet with collaborative teacher teams several hours a week has been invaluable in establishing myself as an instructional leader. It has also given me the opportunity to show my administrative team and teacher leaders what I expect from them. It has also given me the opportunity to see how deeply embedded implicit biases about students are affecting teaching and learning at our school and to begin designing professional development to inspire change. All this would not have been possible in a traditional school schedule when dealing with the normal day to day operations of a school.
2. **Celebrate and collaborate with your team.** When you are a new principal, you have a new team. Even if the team has been established and was working together before your arrival at a school, the team changes with a new leader. I did not have all of the members of my team before I arrived, but there were some folks who had spent the previous year there. One of the most important things that I did was to listen to what they had tried the previous year. This gave me perspective and also helped me approach situations in a way that was more informed. We also had time to meet daily, so we had the opportunity to get to know each other and also collaborate on our shared vision for the school. Lastly, being away from people physically, emphasized the need to celebrate them. I naturally communicate nonverbally and when you are not in the same building as someone it is hard to let them know that you are grateful.

   The school closure forced me to celebrate my staff in writing and verbally and it established a positive culture for our school. It also gave people the opportunity to get to know me and to recognize that my passion for racial equity and social justice is not performative. This recognition may have taken longer if Louisville were not also embroiled in fallout from the murder of Breonna Taylor by the Louisville Metro Police Department; an event that occurred on the last day of in-person school.

1. **Partner with parents.** Shortly after being hired, I received information about the current family involvement at our school. It was disappointing to find out that in previous years, the school and the parents had a contentious relationship and that many of the parents considered the school as elitist and racist. Because, in virtual learning, the parents are teaching students, it is vital for them to be on the same page as the school. Also, when the students are at home and the teachers are not physically with them, daily communication between parents and school staff is more authentic. Throughout the school closure, we were able to establish that we had a primary goal of connecting with families and that the school was a place to get help for anything that they needed to ensure their child's success. We also began a partnership with the National Center for Families Learning who will continue to support us in connecting with our families.
2. **Systems are vital.** With an in-person school, it is easy to get caught up in a reaction loop. You start something and then all of these other things keep popping up. Folks can run down to your office or catch you in the hall and get you off and running on one "emergency" or another. This is impossible when you are in virtual school. The separation requires you to establish systems of functioning. When folks cannot always immediately get ahold of you, they have to have something that they are supposed to do or they will make up their own rules and this can often end in disaster. Being forced to plan ahead, and then when planning for return to school, to outline things ad nauseum so that other people could understand it if I was not available, facilitated the creation of systems that will last and have already improved our school function. Also, establishing common norms, expectations, and systems for rewarding and celebrating students has already begun to address our racial equity goal of increasing our students' sense of belonging.
3. **Make your resources work for you.** Managing financial and human capital are some of the most underrated skills that school leaders must have. In our district, schools had to manage teacher absences internally. Being required to play Tetris with our schedule every time someone was absent, gave us information on skill sets in staff that were previously unknown. There were people at our school who had only done one job the entire time that they had worked there, and the virtual platform and subsequent hybrid model required me to assign them to something else. Even if their placement did not work out, it was a learning experience for all involved. In terms of financial resources, having access to federal

stimulus funds in addition to our school budgets has allowed us to outfit parents and students with things that they needed to make schoolwork for them at home. It has also given us the freedom to use our school-based funds to increase student engagement in new and different ways.

These five lessons in conjunction with starting the year off establishing a common vision for our school's improvement have helped to establish a foundation for the next few years of this turnaround process. If we are to support our students through the compounded obstacles of COVID-19 school closures and navigating a system that has been predicated on some of us winning and some of us losing, we must believe that our students deserve a quality education that pushes them to be independent learners. We must believe that our students and their families want what is best for them. We must believe that all students can learn and perform at high levels, and we must believe that we are the ones who can make these things happen.

REFERENCES

Blasé, J., & Blasé, J. B. (1999). Implementation of shared governance for instructional improvement: Principals' perspectives. *Journal of Educational Administration, 37*, 476–500.

Borman, G. D. (2005). National efforts to bring reform to scale in high-poverty schools: Outcomes and implications. *Review of Research in Education, 29*(1), 1–27. https://doi.org/10.3102/0091732X029001001

Borman, G. D., Hewes, G. M., Overman, L. T., & Brown, S. (2003). Comprehensive school reform and achievement: A meta-analysis. *Review of Educational Research, 73*(2), 125–230.

Dwyer, D. C. (1985). Understanding the principal's contribution to instruction. *Peabody Journal of Education, 63*, 3–18.

Education Endowment Foundation. (2020). *Remote learning, rapid evidence assessment.* London. Education Endowment Foundation. https://educationendowmentfoundation.org.uk/public/files/Publications/Covid19_Resources/Remote_learning_evidence_review/Remote_Learning_Rapid_Evidence_Asses sment.pdf

Education Week. (2021, February 8). *T*he coronavirus spring: The historic closing of U.S. schools (A timeline). *Education Week.* https://www.edweek.org/leadership/the-coronavirus-spring-the-historic-closing-of-u-s-schools-a-timeline/2020/07#:~:text=The%20coronavirus%20created%20mass%20disruption,that%20began%20in%20late%20February

Egelko, B. (2012, January 17). Supreme Court: Schools can't use race to assign students. *SFGATE.* https://www.sfgate.com/bayarea/article/Supreme-Court-Schools-can-t-use-race-to-assign-

2584155.php#:~:text=2007%2D06%2D28%2010%3A,the%20goal%20is%2 0campus%2 0diversity

Feagin, J. (2013). *Systemic racism: A theory of oppression*. Routledge.

Ferguson, P. V. (1896). 163 US 537 (1896). Jurisdiction: United States of America, Supreme Court date of decision, 18.

Hattie, J., & Zierer, K. (2018). *10 mindframes for visible learning: Teaching for success*.

Heck, R. H., & Hallinger, P. (1999). Next generation methods for the study of leadership and school improvement. *Handbook of Research on Educational Administration*, *2*, 141–162.

Holst, J. D. (2020). Toward a Theory of race, change, and antiracist education. *Adult Education Quarterly*, *70*(2), 175–192. https://doi.org/10.1177/0741713619884580

Inoue, A. (2017). Foreword: On antiracist agendas. In F. Condon & V. A. Young (Eds.) *Performing antiracist pedagogy in rhetoric, writing, and communication* (pp. xi-xx). The WAC Clearinghouse

Kentucky Department of Education. (2020, March). *The non-traditional instruction program: Guidance document*.

Latek, T. (2020, June 1). State unemployment rates soar due to COVID-19 pandemic. *Tribune.com*. https://www.thetimestribune.com/news/state-unemployment-rates-soar-due-to-covid-19-pandemic/article_51b6f35e-a1ae-11ea-9a19-f78a6fcec069.html

Leithwood, K., & Duke, D. (1999). A century's quest to understand school leadership. *Handbook of Research on Educational Administration*, *2*, 45–72.

Leithwood, K., Harris, A., & Hopkins, D. (2008). Seven strong claims about successful school leadership. *School Leadership & Management: Formerly School Organization*, *28*, 27–42. https://doi.org/ 10.1080/13632430701800060

Lubienski, S. T. (2002). A closer look at Black-White mathematics gaps: Intersections of race and SES in NAEP achievement and instructional practices data. *Journal of Negro Education*, 269–287.

New Leaders for New Schools. (2009). *Principal effectiveness: A new principalship to drive student achievement, teacher effectiveness, and school turnaround with key insights from the urban excellence framework*.

The New York Times. (2020, April 1). *Kentucky Coronavirus Map and Case Count. The New York Times*. https://www.nytimes.com/interactive/2021/us/kentucky-covid-cases.html

Orfield, G., Mattise, C., Willoughby, B., Anniebrown, & RHforEducation. (2004). *Brown v. Board: Timeline of school integration in the U.S. Learning for Justice*. https://www.learningforjustice.org/magazine/spring-2004/brown-v-board-timeline-of-school-integration-in-the-us. (Formerly Teaching Tolerance, now called Learning for Justice)

Parkerson, D., & Parkerson, J. A. (2014). *Transitions in American education: A social history of teaching*. Routledge.

Plunkett, V. R. (1985). From Title I to Chapter 1: The evolution of compensatory education. *Phi Delta Kappan, 66*(8), 533–537.

Portin, B. S., Knapp, M. S., Dareff, S., Feldman, S., Russell, F. A., Samuelson, C., & Yeh, T. L. (2009). *Leadership for learning improvement in urban schools*. The Wallace Foundation.

Puma, M. J., & Drury, D. W. (2000). *Exploring new directions: Title I in the Year 2000.* https://eric.ed.gov/?id=ED440472

Redding, C., & Nguyen, T. D. (2020). The relationship between school turnaround and student outcomes: A meta-analysis. *Educational Evaluation and Policy Analysis, 42*(4), 493–519. https://doi.org/10.3102/0162373720949513

Smith, W. F., & Andrews, R. L. (1989). *Instructional leadership: How principals make a difference*. Association for Supervision and Curriculum Development.

Thompson, A. (1997). For: anti-racist education. *Curriculum Inquiry, 27*(1), 7–44. http://www.jstor.org/stable/1180053

Tobin, B. (2020, April 16). About 400,000 Kentuckians filed for unemployment over past month due to COVID-19 woes. *Courier Journal.* https://www.courier-journal.com/story/news/2020/04/16/coronavirus-kentucky-116-k-new-residents-file-unemployment/2990017001/

Totenberg, N., & Kaufman, W. (2007, June 29). Supreme Court quashes school desegregation. *NPR.* https://www.npr.org/templates/story/story.php?storyId=11598422

World Health Organization. (2021). *Coronavirus*. https://www.who.int/health-topics/coronavirus#tab=tab_1

EPILOGUE

S. Charles Malka and R. H. Tiell

Reading through some, or all of this book's chapters, you must have noticed the far reaching effects of the COVID-19 pandemic on individuals and organizations alike, and primarily on behaviors at home and at work. Book contributors approached such effects from different angles; drawing on research and their work experience they offered ways to cope with the pandemic's consequences and challenges. In doing so, the authors hope to raise awareness to necessary steps that must be taken to ensure continuation of our daily routines as the pandemic unfolds, and to ensure our preparedness in dealing with future pandemics that are surely to come.

COVID has left deep marks in many areas and affected many lives. Next to the millions who succumbed to the pandemic and those who survived with long-term symptoms, the unfortunate swelling in the ranks of the unemployed is perhaps the second greatest calamity brought about by the virus. The coronavirus has triggered a U.S. employment crisis of epoch proportions, a sudden spiking of unemployment arguably not seen since the Great Depression. Unemployment rates quickly skyrocketed from below 4% to highs approximating 15% by early 2020. And, although the economy was systemically impacted, certain industrial sectors took especially severe hits. These sectors included the airline, cruise and travel related industries; hospitality, events and leisure related; restaurant, dining, and food service related; and sports and entertainment related sectors. Movie theaters, sports arenas, and other event facilities dramatically shut their doors, and many remain in a much reduced or moribund state.

Back to a New Normal: In Search of Stability in an Era of Pandemic Disruption—Insight From Practitioners and Academics, pp. 265–271

The unemployment crisis conflated with other problem areas. Consider, for instance, health concerns for oneself, family members, friends, and coworkers; school interruptions; civil unrest; and even extreme weather conditions. All served to intensify and add an immeasurable sense of anxiety to the unemployment crisis. In some instances, food shortages and problems with the U.S. postal delivery system further added to the core crisis. Prepandemic, many areas around the country viewed the high rates of opioid addiction as a major crisis, and recent reports suggest that opioid addiction has actually worsened as a result of the pandemic. Suffice it to say that there appear to be multiple secondary stressors involved. Among them are disruptions around gender unemployment differences, remote work, work-family balance, childcare, education, and mental health that raises multiple related concerns.

Some of those stressors were addressed in previous chapters of this book calling attention to several leading areas of concern. We touch briefly on those areas and firmly believe that they ought to shape practitioners' intervention agenda for years to come. The sooner policy makers and professionals in relevant fields become cognizant of these areas of concern and their associated effects, the better prepared our communities will be for dealing with future pandemics.

- ***Concerns relative to gender differences***. The pandemic driven economic downturn shows that women have been more adversely affected than men. Two factors seem to have contributed to women being impacted more as the pandemic unfolds. Women tend to be overrepresented in the front line service workers sector leaving them more exposed to the virus and vulnerable to layoffs. Moreover, women still tend to assume more of the childcare and related activities occurring on the home front. During the pandemic that domestic burden has again fallen more to women.
- ***Concerns relative to dual career families***. Dual career couples have been abruptly thrown into a new reality: juggling work and family duties in new ways not previously experienced. This spilled over and called for a redefining of ways for addressing children's needs, caring for aging parents, balancing family and schooling demands, preparing meals, and many related family activities. A new set of stressors occurred which required a whole new reframing of what is meant by work-family balance. Many dual career couples and families have had to reinvent the way the household is managed.
- ***Concerns relative to child and elder care***. Due to the pandemic and many parents' reluctance to keep their children in group settings, many daycare related businesses have shut down temporarily

and others have simply gone out of business. Not having these resources as readily available, childcare responsibilities have inevitably fallen back on parents and grandparents causing much greater stress on the family unit. Parents with disabled children face added challenges. Some parents, often women, have been forced to choose leaving jobs in order to address childcare needs, as well as their children's remote learning needs. The severity and complexity of this secondary stressor is unique to the ongoing pandemic.

- ***Concerns relative to the massive shift to remote work***. Many workplaces were compelled to shift to remote work during the pandemic. Zoom gained new popularity and was quickly adopted by many businesses, professional groups, and individuals as a means of conducting business. Zoom captured the attention of millions of consumers, and Zoom's company growth rapidly caught fire becoming a choice stock purchase. In short order, Zoom and other similar platforms transformed the way the country was doing business. It is generally viewed that this transformation has been so successful that, we are not likely to ever return to a pre-COVID business pattern. Working remotely has not only become increasingly the norm, but it has in turn prompted us to reframe how we think about offices, workplaces and the like. Many employers now recognize that traditional conferences and group meetings that typically involved travel, lodging and related costs can represent significant financial savings when done virtually. Working remotely in turn raised the need for a new employee-employer work contract, as well as concerns about employees feelings of loneliness and social isolation, and particularly about the blurring of work-family lines and balance.
- ***Concerns relative to education and formal learning***. Conventional wisdom has been that recessions customarily contribute to an increase in pursuit of schooling and learning. In other words, a soft job market is generally viewed as an opportune time to upskill, add credentials and strengthen qualifications thereby enhancing one's marketability when the economy turns around. Interestingly enough, we are not witnessing this familiar return to school pattern during the 2020 pandemic. Various factors, many revolving around the virus, appear to be contributing to this change. Some students have been reluctant to return to the college environment until they or their parents see evidence that sufficient safety procedures have been implemented. College faculty and staff have been reluctant to conduct business as usual. Some colleges have had to send students home or revert again to virtual learning. Even when campus safety protocols have been introduced, a sizable number of students and

their parents have instead chosen to attend college closer to home, take a gap year, temporarily abandon study abroad, and in other ways reduce for now the continuation of their prepandemic educational plans. Higher education's inability to ensure the full, traditional "college experience" along with ever increasing college costs and family's anxiety about campus safety have all converged to undercut the pursuit of more schooling or training in this current down economy.

- ***Concerns relative to mental health***. Given the complexity of the 2020 pandemic, one can reasonably assume that mental health challenges have been more severe and have had a deeper impact if only because of the significant number of infections and deaths. Beyond that, the grieving pattern associated with so many people taking sick or worse yet losing spouses, family members, friends, business associates and other loved ones due to the pandemic has likewise taken a much greater toll psychologically.
- ***Concerns relative to negotiating the school to work transition***. Stop and consider, youth are coming into the workforce with relatively little or no prior work experience, they've faced a tighter, weaker job market, and they have entered the workforce with arguably fewer openings, more limited growth potential and weaker prospects for building long range earning power. In recent years, a point that has been repeatedly asserted is that the youthful generations coming along these days stand to not possess the same career opportunities and earning power that their parents had. We now have Generation Z, born after 1996, trying to negotiate their school to work transition. Even in normal times, these transitions can be tricky and filled with uncertainty. Their employment search may be frustrating given the soft labor market. Some will become "boomerangs" by virtue of having to move back in with their parents at least temporarily until they do find employment. Moreover, this transition parallels the time-honored shift from adolescence to adulthood and from dependent to independent status with all its attendant trials and tribulations.

An acute awareness of these areas of concern is essential, but so is being cognizant of the related implications that promise to usher in a new area of undergoing change in the way we conduct ourselves at home, in school, and at work. The profound change in our social behavior and practice is here to stay for a long while, and so are a few pandemic related implications. With work being so central to many individuals and families, and given the accelerated transformation in today's workplace, we identified seven work-related implications that are worthy of mention and are likely to influence service delivery:

- **Remote Work Acceleration:** Perhaps the major overarching work-related feature that has emerged from the 2020 recession is the rapid use of remote work platforms like Zoom. This shift to widescale utilization of such platforms by individuals and businesses alike has quickly become accepted, reliable business practice. Most businesses recognize that this dramatic shift not only saves time and money, but our professional world will continue to push the envelope concerning remote work options and optimization. By the same token, it is generally recognized that there are sizable segments of the population, for example, less advantaged or residents of rural areas, who may lack digital access and thus will be held back. Steps need to be taken to remedy this situation.
- **Virtual Delivery:** Based on the current pandemic reality, based on how the pandemic continues to play out, based on when we ultimately get a widespread vaccinations, and based further on the increased use of remote platforms, we need to be prepared for addressing the above areas of concern in a virtual or hybrid fashion rather than fully live fashion. Initiatives like virtual Career/Job Fairs and specialized long-term unemployment workshops are among the intervention options.
- **Targeted Designs:** Given the more unique nature of the 2020 unemployment scene, whatever assistance is offered will need to be targeted to those industry sectors and populations earlier identified that have been most adversely impacted by pandemic induced unemployment. Once again, these sectors include airline & travel related; hospitality and events related; restaurant, dining and related, sports and entertainment related, and diverse frontline health and emergency services related. This more industry specific approach should pay better return-to-work dividends.
- **Gig Economy:** As earlier indicated, the gig economy typically applies to free lancers, independent contractors, and the contingent workforce. This segment of the workforce has grown exponentially in the last twenty years, It is estimated to now represent a third of the workforce, and it is projected to continue its rapid growth. It has often been termed the "uberization" of the U.S. workforce. Given the gig economy's growth, one can reasonably assume that increasing numbers of younger workers in 2020–2021 are folded into this growth and perhaps even more will do so in years to come.

- **COVID-19 Growth Driven Jobs:** Clyde Christensen has written extensively about "disruptive innovation." The pandemic will likely shake up a number of industry sectors causing accelerated growth of new jobs in some sectors while other industry sectors and occupations retract. In many ways, it's exciting to consider new jobs that may emerge due to the pandemic. Some quick examples include industrial hygiene, virus contact tracers, drone technology, workplace redesigners, and zoom support specialists. Younger individuals in particular are advised to familiarize themselves with COVID driven new fields that are emerging.
- **Alternative Learning and Upskilling:** Although it may not be as much in evidence during this current 2020–2021 recession, there is an old adage that recessionary periods are an opportune time to acquire additional schooling training. Advancing one's knowledge and skills through new learning in order to take advantage of changing workforce demands and trends during a down economy is worth serious consideration. As in-person classes have been curtailed, there has been a corresponding surge in online learning platforms and activities. Recognizing the importance of lifelong learning but needing to conserve financial resources, many individuals are likely to embrace credible, lower cost, short term, stackable badges as a preferred means of upskilling and adding to their credentials and marketability.
- **Bifurcated Recovery Projections**: Lastly, some labor market specialists opine that the economic recovery from the current 2020–2021 recession is likely to take on the form of the capital letter "K." They view this letter K as figuratively capturing the essential bifurcated way they expect this recovery to play out. The top strand of the letter K leaning upward reflects the segment of the population that are more skilled, better educated and more technologically savvy and will therefore land on their feet pretty well. The bottom strand leaning downward reflects the less skilled, more marginally educated segment of the population that will face greater employment challenges. Even as we allow for these possible bifurcated outcomes, a generally long slog to recovery is anticipated.

In closing, *Back to a New Normal* is a book of hope with a positive view of human ingenuity in taming the pandemic, and of human ability to adapt to its severe effects. The world was thrown fast into the pandemic and found itself caught unprepared. With the global economy grinding to a halt, countries are slow to work themselves out of the virus' claws and slow to adjust to necessary changes. The preceding chapters highlight a few of the unfolding changes brought about by COVID-19, and the opportunities that opened up for balancing new rules of behavior within a host of restrictions. The "how-to" strategies that this book contributors offer, may appeal to any reader, but are particularly aimed at practitioners and professionals in various fields, be it supply-chain managers, business leaders, human resource professionals, healthcare specialists, and academic administrators. In preparing this book, our hope is that we were able to make a small contribution by increasing awareness to possible future pandemics that are likely to come, and by proposing practical ways for managing their possible consequences. Whether we succeeded in doing so, is left to the readers of *Back to a New Normal* to decide.

ABOUT THE CONTRIBUTORS

Joanne Rodriguez Addarich, BA, MA, works as an ESL teacher for public school in the state of Kentucky for the past three years. She received a bachelor's degree in education from the University of Puerto Rico, Rio Piedras Campus. She also completed a master's degree in the teaching of English to speakers of other languages at the University of Puerto Rico. Currently, she is working on her final phase of her PhD on Caribbean literature at the School of Humanities, the University of Puerto Rico. Prior to being hired as a teacher for the state of Kentucky, she worked as a middle, public school English teacher in San Juan, Puerto Rico for twenty years. She also worked part time for the Ana G. Mendez College System, at the East University in Carolina, Puerto Rico, as an ESL teacher for four years. She is a proud mother of a daughter and enjoys painting and gardening in her free time. She finds her job very rewarding due to the opportunity it provides to help immigrant families and their children.

L. Craig Austin is an assistant teaching professor in logistics and supply chain management at Florida International University, College of Business. He is also managing director at STS Logistics, in Fort Lauderdale, FL and a registered customs broker. He has more than 30 years in various management roles with organizations in freight forwarding, air and ocean carriers, and trucking operations.

Orville Blackman, PhD, has a dual career as an academic and a consulting specialist in leading organization effectiveness and change management. Dr. Blackman earned a PhD in organizational development and leadership at the University of Louisville. He is a graduate fellow of the National Research Center for Career and Technical Education. The center's research has influenced education, career, training and workforce planning and development policy in the U.S. Departments of Education and Labor. He has published peer review articles and is a keynote speaker at conferences and professional meetings on topics related to organizational effectiveness and innovation, contemporary leadership, labor market demand and supply, international business and cultural awareness, and best practices in talent development and employee performance. He is a certified international business and training program evaluator for the Accreditation Council for Business Schools and Programs. He is also a certified partner of the Predictive Index assessment and a certified diversity, equity, and inclusion specialist. As a consulting specialist in organizational effectiveness, he has significant experience working with complex organizations that are either planning holistic revitalization initiatives or are navigating unplanned change. He has served multinational corporations and Fortune 500 organizations in various industries such as retail, manufacturing and distribution, financial services, health care, publishing, higher education and nonprofit agencies in the United States and the Caribbean. His consulting work includes talent management and optimization, employee learning and development, strategic planning, organizational realignment, executive and leadership coaching, and diversity, equity, and inclusion training. He uses data driven, evidence-based assessments such as the Predictive Index, PXT Select, emotional intelligence and StrengthsFinder. He also uses evidence-based business models such as the Balanced Scorecard, Kotter's Change Model, and Macey and Schneider's Employee Engagement Model to assist organizations in tackling complex issues.

R. Brayton Bowen, AM, SHRM-SCP, is a business consultant, performance coach, author, educator, and professional speaker. He is author of *Recognizing and Rewarding Employees* (McGraw-Hill, 2000). He leads The Howland Group, a strategy consulting and change management firm and is compassion advocate and chief executive officer for Building Better Worlds of Work. His most recent work is *Engaging the Heart for People, Performance, and Profit: Seven Competencies of Compassion@Work* (Building Better Worlds of Work Press, 2020) that increase profit up to 40% and more. His landmark documentary series, "Anger in the Workplace," was aired on public radio nationally in the U.S. A best practice editor and contributing author to the hallmark work *Business* (Bloomsbury Publishing and Perseus Books), he has written for the American Management Association, *HR Magazine* (Society for Human Resource Management) and various other publications. Brayton has been invited to teach at The University of Phoenix, Northwood University and McKendree University. He holds both bachelor's and master's degrees from Brown University. For more information: brayton@buildingbetterworldsofwork.com or brayton@howlandgroup.com; Telephone: 502-558-2154.

Rebecca Carpenter, PhD, is a graduate of Sullivan University in Louisville, Kentucky. She writes about healthcare from her over 40 years of experience as a registered nurse in various aspects of the industry. She continues employment today within a healthcare organization. Rebecca lives in Elizabethtown, Kentucky, with her husband on a 67-acre farm including greenhouses, a vineyard, four rescued horses and several rescued dogs.

Kim Castle, PhD, is an associate professor in the in the Graduate School at Sullivan University. Prior to joining SU, she was an adjunct professor at the University of Pikeville, and the University of the Cumberlands. She specializes in management, entrepreneurship, conflict management mediation, high conflict divorces, and domestic violence. Dr. Castle authored a chapter in L. Wilkin and T. Belak's (2021), *From Discord to Harmony: Making Your Workplace Hum*; she authored *Divorce Bullying—An Epidemic*, published in June 2018 by Balboa/Hay House Press, under the pen name, Twiggy Bean (PhD). And, she presented at Global Business and International Management Conference in Orlando, FL, in 2017. In addition, she often writes articles for her local newspaper, *The Winchester Sun*. Dr. Castle conducts seminars and workshops, teaches the skills to change and motivates clients to seek change. Her philosophy is that "our mistakes do not define us—it is our changes that will be remembered."

Teresa A. Daniel, JD, PhD, serves as dean and professor, Human Resource Leadership Programs at Sullivan University (www.sullivan.edu) based in Louisville, KY. She is also the chair for the HRL concentration in the university's PhD in management program. Dr. Daniel has a significant body of research in HR with an emphasis on two primary areas of inquiry: (1) *counterproductive work behaviors* (focused on workplace bullying, sexual harassment, and toxic leadership), and (2) *Human resources' unique role and its impact on organizational effectiveness* (primarily in the management of toxic workplace emotions, responding to situations of workplace bullying and harassment, dealing with toxic leaders, building positive work cultures, and the management of people during mergers and acquisitions). She provides consulting services focused on these topics at InterConnections (www.interconnectionsllc.com). Dr. Daniel's research has been actively supported by the national Society for Human Resource Management through the publication of numerous articles, interviews, and books. Her newest work is *Organizational Toxin Handlers: The Critical Role of HR, OD, and Coaching Practitioners in Managing Toxic Workplace Situations* (Palgrave Macmillan, 2020). She is also the coauthor of two books with Dr. Gary Metcalf titled *Stop Bullying at Work: Strategies and Tools for HR, Legal & Risk Management Professionals* (SHRM, 2016) and *The Management of People in Mergers & Acquisitions* (Quorum Books, 2001). She has a forthcoming book titled *Guardrails: Taming Toxic Leaders and Building Positive Cultures* (SHRM Books, 2021). Dr. Daniel was honored as an initial fellow of the International Academy on Workplace Bullying, Mobbing, and

Abuse in 2014 and received the *Distinguished Alumnus Award* at Centre College in 2002. Most recently, she was the 2019 grand prize winner of the national *SHRM HR Haiku* contest. She can be reached via email at tdaniel@sullivan.edu or TeresaAnnDaniel@gmail.com.

Michael Hart, EdD, PhD, is an assistant professor at Minnesota State University, Mankato. He has served in several leadership roles in high-tech firms including being a chief executive officer for 12 years. Michael has helped develop and launch three undergraduate computing programs and three graduate programs in disciplines ranging from health informatics to information security. He recently has presented research in the areas of big data systems, computer networks, cybersecurity, distributed and parallel computing, and software development. Michael can be reached at michael.hart-2@mnsu.edu.

J. Claudette Howard, PhD, lives with her family in the southeast region of the United States. She is currently an elementary school principal in an Accelerated Improvement School. In her 18 years as an educator, she has been an elementary school teacher, counselor, and assistant principal, and a middle school assistant principal. Dr. Howard is passionate about social justice and equity in education and is devoted to providing every student with the access and opportunity they need to achieve the excellence they deserve. She is a certified equity literacy facilitator as well as a member of the board of directors for StageOne Family Theater and the Louisville Youth Orchestra. She is also a member of the Diversity, Equity, and Inclusion Committee for the LYO.

Tom G. Javarinis, PhD, CM, LSSBB, is an associate professor at Sullivan University Graduate School. He is married to Angie, and they have three girls: Arielle, Georgette, and Anastasia. Oh! and a six-pound toy poodle named Sofi. Dr. Javarinis has completed several degrees. A bachelor of business administration degree in general management with a minor in accounting from the Detroit College of Business; Dearborn, Michigan. He completed three Master of business Administration degrees from Davenport University: a master's in strategic management with a minor in leadership; a master's in accounting with emphasis on forensics and Fraud; and a master's in healthcare management. Dr. Javarinis also completed his doctor of philosophy degree in general business: organizational behavior and development with a minor in human Resources from Capella University, Minneapolis, MN. His dissertation, "Bipolar Disorder and the Impact it has on a Manager's Career Progression and Leadership Potential" was published and is available on Amazon. Dr. Javarinis also hold various industry certificates: CM - Certified Managers Certificate from the Institute of Certified Professional Managers and James Madison University; Supply Chain Management Certificate from the Supply Chain Management Institute; Lean Six Sigma Black Belt from Management and Strategy Institute; Project Management Certificate from Management and Strategy Institute. Dr. Javarinis has a very simple teaching philosophy which focuses on his role as a mentor/educator and defines what is important about it and involves three principle activities: to continually strive to develop a broad array of teaching skills and adjust them to meet the needs of his students; to truly challenge his students and to evaluate them honestly and fairly; and, to foster student mastery of course material while at the same time helping his students to develop broader, more important skills such as communication and critical thinking. Dr. Javarinis has had the good fortune of working in many different senior management/leadership positions in various industries along with working in Academia for many years both in the online, face-to-face and blended concept. Dr. Javarinis has research interest in the following areas: adaptive learning and technology in the classroom; improving student retention and persistence; effective academic leadership; supporting students who may be at risk of dropping out of college; youth development and how they can be improved, (when, how, and under what conditions); understand and improve the everyday settings of youth in the United States (settings, social environments, boundaries—peers, family, adults); networking, relationships with adults and peers; and opportunities for academic, social, emotional, and identity development; Analyzing personality types and how they assist students (various generational) to ascertain the necessary knowledge, skills, abilities, as well as practical applications for knowing to be successful in their lives

Terry Kibiloski, PhD, has been teaching at the Sullivan University for over 30 years, and has many years of practical experience in leadership, information technology, business, marketing, human resource management, and professional development. In the past, he has worked as a certified public accountant, auditor, computer consultant, business analyst, computer operator, programmer, information technology manager, and project manager. He previously hosted *The Computer Adventure*, a weekly radio show that was featured on the *Louisville Tonight* TV show and was a recurring guest on British and American radio programs. Dr. Kibiloski is a retired U.S. Air Force officer, editor/owner of *Computer Times* (a technology publication in its 30th year), a website developer, marketing consultant, life coach, certified massage therapist, Reiki master, author, and motivational speaker, plus he is working on his second book titled *Lead Yourself to Better Health*, which covers the seven major aspects of life: physical, mental, emotional, spiritual, social, financial, and professional.

Helen MacLennan, MBA, PhD, is an assistant professor of management and the associate department chair of management and operations at Saint Leo University, Donald Tapia College of Business. She holds a BS in business management, an MBA in real estate studies from Marylhurst University, and a PhD in management with a focus in conflict management from Sullivan University. She teaches graduate-level business and doctoral-level research courses and serves on several student dissertation committees. Dr. MacLennan serves on the editorial review board for several academic journals and as a site evaluator for the Accreditation Council for Business Schools and Programs. Her research interests include business management, conflict de-escalation, organizational civility, entrepreneurship, and doctoral credentialing. She has published research in the *Journal of Conflict Management, International Journal of Doctoral Studies, Journal of Excellence in Business Education, Southeast Case Research Journal*, and the *Journal of Transportation Management.*

Shalom Charles Malka, MA, MBA, PhD, is a professor of management at Sullivan University's Graduate School in Louisville, KY. Malka is a former president of numerous franchises in several states, and an acknowledged entrepreneur with extensive work experience in both business and academia for more than three decades. He taught at Haifa University and Ottawa University prior to joining Sullivan University. His teaching and research interests focus on strategy, leadership, human resource management and entrepreneurship. Malka is the author of an eclectic body of research published in peer-reviewed journals, including the *Proceedings of the Academic Organization for Advancement of Strategic and International Studies, Vocational Evaluation and Work Adjustment Association Journal, Journal of Evaluation and Program Planning, Vocational Evaluation and Career Assessment Professionals Journal, Journal of Administration in Social Work,* and *The Journal of Conflict Management.* He earned a BSW from the University of Haifa, an MA from the University of Tel-Aviv, an MBA from Ottawa University, and a PhD from the University of Pittsburgh. He is an active member of the Academy of Management, and a peer reviewer of scientific papers submitted to its entrepreneurship, strategic management, and conflict management divisions' annual meetings. He also serves as a frequent peer reviewer for the *Journal of Career Development.* Malka conducts business valuations pro-bono for small businesses, and serves as a board member of Temple Shalom congregation in Louisville, KY.

Clay Morgan, BA, is an executive director of Business Network International (BNI). He and his team at BNI build powerful networking teams. These networking teams help leaders of small and medium businesses create meaningful connections to grow their businesses. Members of BNI generate millions of referrals and billions of dollars in revenue for each other every year. In 2020 alone, that was over $17.5 billion. With 17 years in the industry, and 8 years as executive director of BNI, Clay has been a leader locally and globally within the BNI community. Among his other roles, he is serving as chairman of BNI's U.S. franchise advisory council, and a member of The Founder's Circle. Clay has received various awards for excellence in performance and operations, including recognition as a member of BNI's Mastery Circle and Platinum Club. He is a graduate of the University of Kentucky with a BA in integrated strategic communications and political science.

Anthony Piña, MS, EdD, is associate provost for teaching and learning at Sullivan University, where he oversees online learning, faculty development and general education. He has been a consultant to Fortune 500 corporations, small businesses, local government agencies, nonprofit organizations, the U.S. Department of Defense and numerous educational institutions across the country. Tony has developed and taught various online courses and developed online degrees from the associates to the doctorate. He has published 6 books and more than 70 academic and scholarly publications on online/distance education, educational technology, and management.

Bob H. Tiell, MA, career and vocational consultant, at the Psychology Resource Group. Bob Tiell has been a leading professional in the delivery of career services in the Louisville region for many years. As former director of JFCS' Career & Workforce Development division, he created, led and managed the delivery of a wide range of career and workforce development services to the entire community. Bob is a change agent. For individual clients, services include career assessment and management, career coaching and strategizing, college and school advisement, vocational evaluation, employment counseling, and various other career, schooling, and professional development services. For attorneys, Bob qualifies as a vocational expert and conducts vocational evaluations to assess employability and earning power. For organizational clients, services include personnel screening, outplacement, team building, executive coaching, family business consulting, assessment of "hi-pots" and other consulting services. Bob and his team also historically launched and led several projects, workshops, and seminars revolving around career and workforce development issues. Bob is also a Louisville Leadership Center alum. Beyond pioneering delivery of career and college advisement services, Bob and his team, in the spirit of social entrepreneurship, launched several other innovative programs over the years. They include the first SAT Prep. Class, Job Club, Navigate Enterprise Center (business start-ups), a family business center, and our community's first "brain gain" initiative. Special projects include the national award-winning long-term unemployment project representing collaborations with other community-based organizations. Business First also recognized Bob as a top local career specialist. Bob's background and training in the behavioral sciences, assessment, higher education, rehabilitation, business, and workforce areas makes him highly qualified to assist clients on a variety of career, schooling, talent, performance, and workforce development issues. He can be reached at 502-445-5183, 502-394-9990, and bhtiell@gmail.com

LaVena Wilkin, PhD, is the director of PhD programs and graduate management programs at Sullivan University. Before joining Sullivan, she spent 26 years in the construction industry, and 3 of those years she co-owned a masonry subcontracting company. Dr. Wilkin has facilitated workshops on communication, conflict, emotional intelligence, forgiveness, P.E.A.C.E. from Conflict, and workplace bullying for the Center for Non Profit Excellence, The Archdiocese of Louisville, Integrating Women Leaders, FireKing, Governor's Equal Employment Opportunity Annual Conference, the Academic Leadership Academy, the Society for Strategic Human Resources Managers, Unity of East Louisville, Duke Energy, and several other organizations. She also created a basic conflict management course for the Collaborative Institutional Training Initiative.

Dr. Wilkin published an article on workplace bullying in the International Journal of Business and Social Science, and for several years she wrote a quarterly column for *Business First*. She contributed a chapter in *The Handbook of Mediation: Research, Theory, and Practice*. She is also coeditor of a book entitled *Organizational Conflicts: Challenges and Solutions*. She is the editor for the *Journal of Conflict Management*, a scholarly journal that publishes research in many of the multidisciplinary areas of managing conflicts. She co-edited a book, entitled *From Discord to Harmony: Making the Workplace Hum*, which was published in March 2020. In addition, her latest project, *The Handbook of Organizational Conflict Management,* should be available through De Gruyter, publishing in February 2022. She is a certified mediator, conflict coach and employee engagement facilitator. Dr. Wilkin earned her bachelors and master's degrees from Sullivan University. She earned her PhD in conflict analysis and resolution from Nova Southeastern University in Ft. Lauderdale, Florida. Her dissertation topic was workplace bullying in academe. Dr. Wilkin is the vice-president emeritus for the board of directors at Unity of East Louisville. Additionally, she previously served on the board of directors for the Society for the Prevention and Aggression Among Adolescence.